PHYSICIAN WEALTH MANAGEMENT MADE EASY

HOW TO BUILD AND PROTECT
YOUR WEALTH IN UNCERTAIN TIMES

Physician
Wealth
Management
Made Easy

MICHAEL ZHUANG

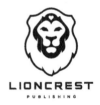

LIONCREST
PUBLISHING

PHYSICIAN WEALTH MANAGEMENT MADE EASY

How to Build and Protect Your Wealth in Uncertain Times

ISBN   978-1-61961-792-6   *Paperback*

978-1-61961-793-3   *Ebook*

Contents

Introduction

Twelve years ago, I got a call from my internist.

"Michael, I'm afraid I can't be your doctor anymore," he said, right after hello.

It was an odd opening, and his voice sounded strained. Doc Johnson and I had always been on friendly terms. Had I done something to offend him?

"What's going on, Doc?" I replied. "Is it…is it my insurance?"

"No, Michael," he said and took a deep breath. "I've been diagnosed with pancreatic cancer. And…" He paused again. "I have only a few months to live."

"Wow, that's terrible, Doc."

I didn't quite know how to go on and ask, "OK, but why did you call *me*? I'm no doctor. What can *I* do about it?" So I just waited on the line.

At last, Doc Johnson continued. "Michael, my family's totally unprepared for this, not just emotionally, but... financially. I'm sorry, but I had to call, because you're the only financial guy I know. Can you give us some advice? Help us figure this out?"

Now, at this point in my life, I was not a financial planner, and I had never been a financial planner. I was a numbers guy, not a people guy. Since college, I had worked in major trading houses. And just then, I was the owner of my own hedge fund—a very successful hedge fund in which I worked with only a handful of wealthy investors.

Most days, I never spoke to a soul, not even about money. I simply sat in front of computer screens up in my Florida beach condo, watching the digits roll over, as beautifully as the surf.

But how could I refuse a man who was about to die?

"Well, sure, Doc," I said, finally pulling my eyes away from my trading program. "I'll take a look at least."

Two days later, I found myself at Dr. Johnson's house, meeting his family.

The house was lovely and large, as befitted a busy internist. But Mrs. Johnson was so distraught that she actually looked sicker than her husband and so weak she could barely speak. The eyes of their teenage daughter had grown red and swollen from days of crying. The parents had not yet given the news to their son, at college in California. They weren't sure if they should pull him out of school in the middle of his semester to come help out.

I took a deep breath and told these heartsick people to go through their desks and closets and pull out all their legal and financial papers. These papers were, indeed, in a total mess.

I was shocked to see that such a solid man of science and precision as Doc Johnson was that he had no idea how to handle money. Little by little, I realized not only had he made some poor investments, but he was also heavily in debt.

The good doctor had only $200,000 in savings, mostly in cash at a bank earning nothing. After many years in his beautiful house, he still carried a $1 million mortgage. He had no succession plan for his practice. And, because he had no business overhead insurance, he would have to personally bear the costs of shutting down that practice.

I spent three months helping the Johnson family get organized, rethink their expenses, and prepare for the inevitable. And when my internist passed away, I stayed on board to help his wife and kids make the necessary financial transition and adjustment.

From my point of view as a "financial guy," their situation was not at all dire. They did have to move out of the big house, but they found something smaller and maybe more comfortable, right nearby. Equity from the sale of their big house paid off the mortgage and left a nice bonus. Mrs. Johnson did have to go back to work as a nurse, but perhaps that helped keep her mind off the loss of her husband. By the time the dust settled, the Johnson family had about $700,000 invested in a diversified portfolio with an expected 7 percent return at manageable risk.

One day, when I was meeting with Mrs. Johnson, she suddenly reached out, gave me a big hug, and said, "Michael, how can I thank you enough? I wouldn't have known how to handle all this without your help."

Now, I had not made a dime out of helping the Johnsons. I had done it all as a favor. But I felt more rewarded from that hug and her words of gratitude than from any hundreds of thousands of dollars made by split-second trading on the stock exchange.

I realized I had made a big difference in the lives of good people. I had helped a man who had helped other people his whole career. And for the first time in my life, I felt that my financial talents were actually needed—that my work could have meaning.

It took me a year to fully transform my hedge fund into a financial advisory focused on physicians (in fact, I never even changed the name). But it was the best decision I ever made.

A COMMON THEME

Once I started down my new path, I began to talk to dozens of physicians of all kinds, and I found that Doc Johnson's chaotic financial situation was quite common. I'd do what I called discovery interviews, which means I'd invite a doctor out for coffee just to tell me confidentially about his or her financial life. I had to work hard to convince these nice people I wasn't trying to sell them anything.

"What's your biggest challenge?" I'd ask. "How do you make your practice pay?"

I think these doctors really enjoyed having someone listen to their money headaches—at least, once they realized I wasn't trying to trick them into some bogus get-rich-quick scheme or pull them into yet another costly insurance policy. Indeed, I learned that these physicians hear from financial salesmen nearly every week.

What did I find? Again and again, some of the smartest, most educated, most methodically trained professionals in our society said to me, "Listen, Michael, I'm making good money, but I am not on top of my personal finances. I don't have time. I don't know what I'm doing. And I'm making a mess of it."

Doc Johnson died in 2006. In the years since, and after talking to hundreds of doctors in every imaginable specialty and situation, I have found that a shocking number are in seriously poor fiscal shape. Only a tiny percentage can even explain their financial planning out loud, much less with confidence.

Not surprisingly, perhaps, I've also learned that not all doctors end up wealthy.

Even when earning $300,000, $400,000, $500,000, or more a year, many hardworking physicians have little left when December 31 rolls around.

SAVVY DOCS?

Which docs handle money best?

You might think that physicians who go into private practice would be the most savvy in personal finance. Certainly, they make the most money. But because they're out on their own and do not have larger organizations to help impose financial discipline on their practices or their retirement plans, doctors with their own offices often get into the most trouble.

Why? For starters, a large influx of money can bring with it overconfidence and a lack of care with cash. But more importantly, these folks focus so narrowly on building their practices that little time and energy remain for thinking about tax planning and long-game stock portfolios.

Physicians in private practice are certainly the worst at planning for retirement. Many private practitioners have not built up a nest egg or made the necessary investments during their prime years of practice. Now, they find themselves in their sixties with no plan for the succession of their carefully built businesses. Often, private practitioners end up working until age seventy or seventy-five, when they would much rather be lounging on a beach.

By contrast, doctors who work for hospitals or other large

organizations usually have some kind of retirement plan laid out for them. Some even earn pensions. And because during their career their income arrives in a more predictable and constrained fashion, they may better limit their own expenses. The result? Even though doctors in corporate practice may not have earned as much over the years as doctors in private practice, when it comes time to retire, they often find themselves in better shape.

Such are the ironies that pursue even the most successful physicians, across all specialties.

WHO SHOULD READ THIS BOOK?

If you are a young physician, you can make financial mistakes and still recover. If you are mid-career or late-career, you may have little chance to bounce back from unforced errors. Either way, I've written this book to give you a physician-centric view of personal finance.

Some of the information here will apply to only those in private practice, but most sections will apply equally to doctors working in clinics and hospitals.

Much of what I discuss will also apply to dentists and other clinicians, although thanks to the regulatory and legal environment, practicing MDs see the greatest financial challenges.

A WORD TO THE SKEPTICAL PHYSICIAN

I have found that doctors are more skeptical than most people about financial advisors—and about books such as this one.

I'm sure this skepticism arises partly from the confusing licensing standards for financial advisors, along with the lack of strict educational standards. Doctors, after all, are highly educated, rigorously trained, and carefully licensed.

Then there's the "salesperson problem." As we shall see in later chapters, only about 7 percent of financial advisors operate on a fee-only basis. The other 93 percent of "advisors" are actually salespeople.

Doctors have learned to spot disguised salespeople a mile away—or at least down a long hospital hallway. They often find themselves specially targeted by people peddling dubious investments: everything from real estate speculations to self-dealing insurance schemes to obscure financial vehicles.

But it also may be that doctors just have a hard time accepting advice from other kinds of professionals—ever.

I can't help but give you an example from my own experience.

I once proposed a portfolio to a potential client who was

a prominent surgeon. It was a highly diversified portfolio using five asset-class funds. One was a fund that literally invested in the entire US stock market. Another was an international fund with a large basket containing *all* publicly traded international stocks. The third was a real estate fund that encompassed *all* real estate-related investment vehicles around the globe. The fourth was a corporate bond fund investing in *all* corporate bonds. Finally, there was a government bond fund investing in *all* government bonds.

The surgeon looked at this portfolio with deep skepticism. Why? Because it had only five funds, whereas another financial advisor had created a portfolio that contained a hundred different stock-picking mutual funds. My client told me how diversified this other portfolio would be, compared with mine.

I raised my eyebrows and smiled. Then I tried to explain that my five funds were actually far more diversified, because the person running each of those hundred mutual funds might choose to pick only a small number of stocks in a narrow class—for example, big-cap US stocks. Indeed, every one of those hundred funds might have the *same* few stocks in them. Every single mutual fund, for example, might contain AIG. This was not diversification.

Just as importantly, actively managed mutual funds tend to

have high expense ratios. Many of them carry as much as a 7.5 percent load. (*Load* is financial jargon describing the money a mutual fund company takes from your account to pay a broker for directing your money to the fund company.) All five funds I proposed were no-load funds with very low expense ratios—as they were asset-class funds, not stock-picking funds.

This otherwise very wise surgeon would not listen to me. He told me he wanted only US stocks, because US stocks had done well the year before. He would not believe that international stocks might do well in the next year, as they had done poorly in the previous year.

I tried to explain that the previous year's performance does not predict the following year's performance. One should never use past returns to anticipate future returns; indeed, you will find that very warning printed on any investment report.

In short, this fine doctor was cocksure about his own diagnosis and prognosis. He trusted his judgment over mine, even though I do this every day; even though he had little experience in my "branch of medicine;" and even though he had never made a personal study of investment science (and yes, I do think it's a science, as I will discuss in Chapter 5).

He was looking for someone to affirm his thinking, rather

than give him advice. Unfortunately, his thinking was entirely wrong.

Why did the prominent surgeon trust his own opinion over mine? Not because he was foolish, but because in his daily practice, he had learned to trust his own opinion over that of others, time and time again.

No doubt, in his own realm, this doctor *was* usually right, even when others disagreed.

Could I have won him over by playing along with his self-destructive instincts? Probably. But personally, I refuse to do that. I will only take a client when I can add substantial value to their lives.

In this case, that would have been impossible.

A WORD TO THE SAVVY—AND THE FEARFUL

On the other hand, I know some doctors who are highly schooled in finance, who would have instantly accepted my advice about diversification. Indeed, one of the best books ever written about investing came from the famous William "Bill" Bernstein, a neurologist.

If you are a financially savvy doctor, the advice in my book may at first seem elementary. But I hope my book will help you look at the biggest possible picture—and lead you to examine your overall personal financial structure. Are you thinking about planned charitable giving, protecting your heirs, creating a succession plan for your practice, or protecting your assets from predators?

It's important to approach financial planning not as mere *investing* but as comprehensive *wealth management.* In these pages, you will get a full overview of wealth management as it plays out through a medical career. Your goal: Ensure that you build yourself a solid financial structure at each stage of your working life.

That said, in Chapter 5, we will go deeply into a peer-reviewed, clinically tested investment theory that should please the most rigorous and knowledgeable of medical researchers.

If you are *not* financially savvy, if you usually find yourself fearful of personal finance, or if you believe the subject is somehow beyond you, this book has been designed to give you new confidence, as well as a solid basis for getting your entire financial house in order.

I've done my best to keep it short, straightforward, and jargon-free.

THE FINANCIAL LIFE CYCLE OF A PRACTICING PHYSICIAN

Each phase of a doctor's career includes its own financial challenges. Or, maybe we should call them "hazards."

Later, I will give you a number of cautionary tales from my experience with clients. For now, let's explore the typical life cycle of a physician's career.

EARLY THIRTIES: THE CAREER BEGINS

Doctors begin earning a serious income much later than most people, even highly educated people. You have to complete four to five years of pre-med work in college, four years of medical school, and then three to seven years of residency, depending on your specialty. That's potentially between eleven and sixteen years of little or no earnings. By the time you're in a position to make a substantial income, you're likely in your thirties with a family to feed.

Doctors set out with fewer earning years ahead of them, and this late start also includes a hidden danger. Let's call it pent-up monetary frustration, or PMF. No doubt, you can find this condition well described in a medical journal somewhere.

Let me tell you about a young doctor of my acquaintance, whom I will call Rajesh.

Rajesh completed his residency in oncology at age thirty-five, and straightaway, he landed a job with a big hospital in Washington, D.C. Because of his high-demand specialty, his starting salary was $350,000 a year.

Now, up until that moment, Rajesh had never earned more than $50,000 in any one year. He had been living in a tiny apartment with his girlfriend, where the two of them consumed large quantities of lentil soup and potatoes. He owned a beat-up Chevy, but he usually rode his bicycle to work to save on gas.

By age thirty-five, Rajesh was suffering from an acute case of PMF. The symptoms were ready to break out all over.

Sometime just after Rajesh received his first huge paycheck, he came to talk to me about what he called "investments"—even though he as yet had virtually *no* money in the bank, and he owed about $300,000 in student loans. He didn't want to know about stock funds; he wanted to know how to finance the very large house he wanted to buy. He also talked about a new, shiny black BMW he had seen at a dealership.

In short, Rajesh really, *really* wanted to start spending money.

Our meeting took place in his apartment, which looked

pretty much like a dorm room in Sparta—no decorations on the walls and thrift store furniture. I asked him, "Are you comfortable with this lifestyle?"

"Perfectly comfortable," he said, shrugging. "But hey, listen. In just a few years—maybe five—they say my salary should go up to $450,000, even $500,000." Then he went back to discussing five-bedroom houses and the BMW 5 Series.

"So, Rajesh," I interrupted, "are you aware that $350,000 a year puts you into the highest federal income tax bracket, which means the IRS will want 35 to 39 percent of your salary? Also, in D.C., the district taxes run sky-high, maybe 8 to 10 percent on top of the feds. So, your marginal income tax rate overall will be close to 50 percent, even though not all of the $350,000 will be subject to this 50 percent tax. You should expect to pay maybe 35 percent in taxes, or a third of your income."

I hated to see the glow on his face fade, but it's my job to speak truth to fantasy.

"That leaves you with $220,000 to $240,000, depending. From that, you have to pay the loan service on your student debt—I'm guessing about $15,000 a year. Your living expenses are going to go up, even if you don't buy a house, and you may well decide to marry your lovely girlfriend and have a few kids. You are, after all, already thirty-five."

But I wasn't quite done. "You also live in a time of great political uncertainty in regard to health care. You believe you will be earning $500,000 in five years, but truly, none of us can reliably predict the earning power of doctors, even a short time from now."

Indeed, young doctors face the most uncertainty from possibly radical changes in the overall health-care delivery system. Sometimes, these physicians have been inspired by parents who also practiced medicine, but the young docs are entering a career that has become far riskier than anything their parents faced. I'll talk in detail about these "macro challenges" in Chapter 1. But the bottom line? These challenges demand caution.

By the end of our meeting, I had told Rajesh that instead of thinking about purchasing a fancy house and car, he should focus on accumulating assets to invest for the future. I explained to him how capital gains are taxed at a much lower rate than income earned from labor, so he should focus on becoming a man of means, earning those capital gains year in and year out.

"And remember that you will *never* have to impress people with your *wealth*; they will already admire you as a doctor, regardless of the size of your house. Your top financial priority should be building up to a $1 million asset base, which you can then invest and grow over time. Do that," I said, "before you buy a shiny black BMW."

FORTIES AND FIFTIES: MID-CAREER STRESS

A physician at mid-career faces a whole new set of challenges. Often, these are self-created.

Let me tell you about Dr. Edwards, a wonderful ENT who came to me for help a few years ago. At age forty-five, Dr. Edwards had been in practice for just over a decade, and he had his own private office with a couple of assistants; the practice netted him about $450,000 a year.

The good doctor also owned a massive house on a large piece of land. Indeed, you might call it a mansion on a farm. It was just the kind of mansion that all doctors desire, and it was presided over by his wife, who did not work but devoted herself to raising their two lovely daughters. The daughters attended the very best private high school in the area. To the outside world, he appeared to have the perfect life.

Unfortunately, to Dr. Edwards, it did not seem so perfect. When he first came to me for advice, he said that he woke up every day with tremendous stress and went to bed every night suppressing panic attacks.

You see, he knew that although he was earning a lot of money, he was saving almost none of it. After ten years of practice, Dr. Edwards had put aside only about $200,000 in savings and investments.

How was that possible? Well, the mortgage and upkeep on his house and land was enormous. Then there were the tuitions for the girls and the leases on his and his wife's no-doubt shiny black BMWs. There was the debt service on his student loans and the $40,000 a year he paid for malpractice insurance.

Part of Dr. Edwards's stress came from the enactment of the Affordable Care Act (ACA), also known as Obamacare. Obamacare seemed to upend just about everything the doctor knew about the business of medicine, and it seemed to increase the risk on just about everything he did.

The legislation did not actually harm his business economically—as he later discovered—but coping with the required paperwork and changes just about sent him to the ER as a patient, not a doctor. No doubt the planned repeal of the ACA has him just as worried.

Earlier, I said that the greatest impact of political change around health care will hit younger physicians. But the *stress* of change may be higher for mid-career physicians who see their business models undermined again and again just when their own career options have become more limited. A younger colleague may easily shift to a career in, say, medical technology. That's a tough move for a forty-five-year-old.

When we met, Dr. Edwards was not, unfortunately, stressed about the way he had invested his $200,000—which he had sunk into an expensive life insurance product sold to him by a "friend" in the insurance business. Each year, he pushed another $40,000 into that plan.

When I explained to the doc that this insurance policy made little or no sense as an investment strategy, his shoulders sagged. "So, what you're telling me," he said, "is that if I continue on this path, I'm going to work myself to death, and I still won't have enough to retire comfortably?"

"Perhaps we can change your path," I offered.

I worked with Dr. Edwards for several years. I began by replacing his "whole life" insurance with a number of laddered "term life" insurance policies with terms ranging from five years to twenty years. The reasoning? By year twenty, his wealth should grow to about $6 million—when he could die without his wife and daughters going hungry.

We also agreed that he should put aside at least $120,000 each year. Sure enough, with a few lifestyle changes, including downsizing after his daughters went to college, his asset base has grown to about $1.5 million after six years. He also has an asset target. When he gets to $3 million, he's going to slow down. He may still work, but he will work less.

Eventually, Dr. Edwards *will* be able to retire.

I wish I could say that about all the physicians I know.

RETIREMENT

Many doctors have spent their whole lives—often right back to childhood—planning for a career in medicine. They plotted their high school science courses, agonized over their college curriculum, lined up their references, and charted every step of med school and beyond.

But few seem to do much planning for retirement. Few seem to have a solid succession plan for their private practices. And even fewer have paid attention to the proper accumulation and investment of their wealth—or the financial discipline needed during one's career to ensure a comfortable retirement.

I know a plastic surgeon who earns in the neighborhood

of $1 million a year, but at age sixty, he has not built up a fortune. Instead, he has built a lifestyle that costs him $500,000 a year. If he stopped working tomorrow without changing that lifestyle, he would enjoy it for just one or two years before going bankrupt.

I once asked this surgeon if he felt his quality of life was ten times higher than it was when he was making only $50,000 a year during his residency. His answer? "I don't feel much different at all. Honestly, I just don't know where my money goes." Then he thought of one place the money went. "Just the other day, I did buy a $2,000 outfit for my wife. It's still hanging in her closet—she's had no occasion to wear it."

I set up an automatic "wealth builder" system for this fine surgeon. That's a program that automatically moves $20,000 from his bank account to his investment account and invests the money every month. If he doesn't see the money, I figure he won't have the urge to spend it.

The Crucial Role of Succession Planning

Another client of mine nurtured a highly successful Ob-Gyn practice with thousands of patients. His office generated $2 million to $3 million in revenues each year. Unfortunately, as he neared retirement, he had made no plan whatsoever for the sale or transition of his practice. In the end, he just gave it away to his associate doctors and received literally nothing from the equity he had created. With the proper arrangements, he should have been able to leave with at least $1 million from the sale of his practice, perhaps more. However, he simply never investigated the possibility or did the groundwork for such a sale.

Fortunately, this gynecologist had his other finances in order, and with my investment help, he was able to maintain much of his lifestyle after he retired. But I see succession mistakes made by older doctors again and again. They simply fail to understand the issues, and *they wait too long.*

In Chapter 4, we'll discuss planning for the succession of a private practice. For now, let me say that succession cannot be planned just a few months before retirement or even just a year before.

In fact, most experts estimate that it takes five full years of planning and transition to maximize the return on a successful practice. The best strategy is usually to work out an internal transition in which you bring in an associate doctor to whom you can eventually sell your equity. This takes time. You cannot just go to an associate doctor one day and say, "I'd like to sell you my part of the practice for $2 million." They may not have the money, and it might not make sense for them if the plan was not in the works for some time.

As we shall see, taking succession steps early can also improve your working life right away.

The Crisis of the Aging Physician

Many doctors wish they could retire but find they cannot. Indeed, thanks to the macro stresses I discuss in Chapter 1, more and more doctors wish they could retire early.

Unfortunately, because of an expensive lifestyle and poor planning, doctors often find themselves practicing to age seventy, even seventy-five. They do this more out of necessity than from an abiding love of medicine. Often, they practice until they have a hard time moving around the office or the hospital.

As these physicians age, their risks increase, especially their risk of lawsuits. Why? Not because older doctors are less competent, but simply because the lawyers for plaintiffs think that older doctors have more money. Younger doctors make just as many mistakes, but they have less assets to attack.

I don't need to tell you that the great majority of medical

lawsuits are without merit. And lawsuits against older doctors have no more merit than those against their younger colleagues.

Electronic Medical Records Overwhelm

The advent of massive electronic medical records (EMR) systems has also pushed more and more older doctors to seek retirement. Often, physicians find themselves caught between a rock and a hard place. On the one hand, they need to keep working because they did not plan and save. On the other hand, they are ill-adapted to new computerized systems and reporting demands.

The media have done a poor job of reporting on the stress and burden of new EMR requirements, especially the burden coming as a result of the ACA.

The Obamacare mandate included a drive to record *everything* in medical health records. The idea, of course, was to ensure that records could be easily shared among different doctors. But the unintended consequences have been huge.

For starters, a lot of older doctors are simply not comfortable working with complex computer software. In the past, they would just see a patient and then record their diagnosis on paper. Now, they have to input massive quantities of data into the EMR system in a fixed format. One of my doctor clients, for example, says he sees patients for about eight hours every day, and then he spends another three hours inputting their medical information into an EMR system.

Politicians and laypeople may find it hard to believe this burden would cause a doctor to seek retirement, but there's actual data to show that the EMR burden is causing doctors to *commit suicide* in increasing numbers.

How is that possible?

Doctors are typically idealistic men and women who have spent their lives preparing to help others. They find meaningful, rewarding work in seeing patients. Inputting data often seems valueless, even dangerous. Miscoded procedures can become evidence in court for malpractice lawsuits or even criminal proceedings for Medicare fraud.

Even accurately recorded notes may simply make it easier for an opposing lawyer to establish a trail of potentially actionable decisions by the doctor—just one more way to find fault.

Many, many older physicians have grown to hate data input with a passion. It's causing many to burn out—and yes, consider suicide. I don't mean to be facetious, but doctors are very good at killing themselves. Health-care professionals show a much higher rate of success in their suicides than the general population.

Younger physicians may find data input a burden, but they have grown up with this necessity. They're better at understanding computers, and they simply have more stamina for late hours in front of the screen.

I have no doubt that EMR offers great value to society. A meaningful record of previous tests, medications, and outcomes that can move from doctor A to doctor B no doubt saves lives. And EMR can save money, because redundant tests, even redundant questioning, can be avoided.

But the systems have not been well designed. Systems from office to office don't "talk" to each other properly—meaning that doctor B can't always get the information from doctor A in a timely or useful format. Part of the problem arises from our nation's deep belief in capitalism, which means the government has been reluctant to enforce a single standard. Instead, it allows software vendors to fight among themselves over how to store and present data.

The result? Cascading technology and data issues exist through the whole medical industry; good intentions, poor execution.

From a financial perspective, the cost burden on doctors adds greatly to the overall stress equation. Doctors and their staffs must spend serious time and money just implementing and training on all these different technologies. And doctors may have to employ a "medical scribe" to follow them around and record everything they do and say. Such scribes introduce even more issues, because many doctors, especially older doctors, do not trust the scribe's accuracy. If a scribe writes something wrong in a medical system, it can be good material for a future lawsuit—or worse.

Moving Out of Private Practice

Many overburdened, aging physicians in private practice have been considering selling out to a larger medical group and working for a paycheck. These larger groups can better cope with the raft of new technological and legal issues introduced by the ACA and other changes in medicine. But it's hard for an older physician, accustomed to being his or her own boss, to make the transition to become an employee. It may feel humiliating after a lifetime of independence, and the loss of freedom may be substantial.

Many an older physician has sold his or her practice to a large medical group only to tell me, "I screwed up. I never should have done it. The guy running this big group is no doctor; he's an MBA. He really knows nothing about medicine, and he cares only about the bottom line. The administration tells us what to do based on profitability, not medical necessity. I wish I could get out of this situation."

Doctors make this complaint often enough to cause deep reservations among others considering the move.

AFTER RETIREMENT

The retired physician does not have to face all the changes going on in the medical profession, but new challenges arrive in every phase of life. The challenges of retirement grow increasingly larger for all of us, thanks in part to the increased longevity created through the advancement of medicine itself.

I would venture to say, however, that doctors have a tougher challenge than most. Why? Because despite their position among the highest earners in American society, the number of doctors who enter retirement with high levels of debt and unsustainable lifestyle trends is much higher than the number in the general population of "the wealthy."

The Doctor's House

For some reason, these unsustainable lifestyles often come from *housing*. Doctors, as a class, seem to enjoy buying and owning houses they can't really afford.

I met with one cardiologist who had just retired at age seventy-five. He had about $3 million put aside, which one might consider is a very tidy sum. But he was spending $20,000 a month to sustain his lifestyle. How was that possible? Well, he had somehow accumulated three residences, and they each cost serious money.

Besides his home in Orlando, the cardiologist had purchased a vacation house on the coast, and he was renting an expensive condo in Manhattan. Why? So he could spend more time with his children, who all worked in and around New York. Between the mortgages, the rent, the property taxes, and the upkeep, he was spending $17,000 a month just on housing. Only $3,000 a month went to everything else in his life. Indeed, like my young doctor friend, he was probably eating a lot of potatoes and lentil soup.

With $3 million in retirement assets properly invested, this successful physician could have lived on $10,000 a month forever. But at $20,000 a month, his nest egg would not sustain him for the rest of his life.

When we sat down together and did the math, I asked him, "Tell me, what do you enjoy most in life?"

"I love jazz," he said. "I love to go to jazz bars and listen to the best players."

When I asked him how much he budgeted for jazz bars, he said, "About $200 a month." In other words, he spent $200 a month on what he really loved and $17,000 a month to maintain three houses. Not only that, but the maintenance and hassles associated with these three houses were greatly adding to his overall stress; they were meant to make him happy, but they were making him miserable.

Doctors often have multiple residences. They'll own a home, a vacation cottage, an investment property, and a house they buy in advance for their retirement residence. They may think such properties make good investments, but more often, they become a liability and do not pencil out over time. If you live in a house one-third of the year, but you have to pay $5,000 a month for mortgage and upkeep, the math can work against you, even with the appreciation of the property year to year.

More importantly, perhaps, your energy goes into something that is not your life's focus and expertise.

Charitable Planning

Retirement offers opportunities beyond lowering stress and enjoying the things you love.

Once my retired physicians have stabilized their finances,

they often turn to me for advance charitable planning. They are usually thrilled to find this as a real possibility for their later years. As practicing physicians, these folks have had a meaningful impact on the lives of others, and they want to continue to make an impact in retirement.

First, however, they must get control over their basic finances. Even the wealthy cannot give attention to their charitable inclinations if they live in financial uncertainty.

MY ROLE AND THE ROLE OF THIS BOOK

Earlier, I spoke about the skepticism doctors seem to have for professionals in financial planning. Perhaps I can ease some of the skepticism and open you to the rest of this book with an analogy to good medical practice.

Suppose you were a family practitioner, and during a series of routine tests, you thought you heard something odd in my electrocardiogram. Then you read my blood tests and saw that my lipid profile was off the chart and my cholesterol was extremely high.

At that point, you would probably not say, "I am going to treat this man myself." You would probably send me to a cardiologist.

You would recognize that different fields of medicine require different expertise.

I have a different field of expertise than yours, but I see my financial advisor role as somewhat similar to that of a family practitioner. I stay in touch with my clients on a regular basis. I do regular financial checkups in which I take their vitals and do some tests. I help plan my clients' investments. And yes, just like a family doctor, I might advise them to eat less fatty foods and "exercise" their investments more effectively.

But if I find a serious issue with their taxes or their estate planning—or if they face a significant legal issue—I do not try to solve all their problems on my own. I refer them to my network of experts. I find them a good tax accountant, a reliable estate attorney, or a winning litigation lawyer. I get them the right specialist, and we all stay in touch on the problem.

Like a responsible doctor, I know the vital role played by referrals.

WHAT IS A FINANCIAL ADVISOR?

In spite of my personal, medically flavored definition of the term, I realize that the role of financial advisor is not well defined by our society in general. You will find financial advisors, financial planners, investment advisors, and wealth advisors who are actually insurance salespeople, annuity salespeople, or stockbrokers.

Later, we'll talk about how to interview and select a financial advisor. But for now, be warned that all these titles are merely hats anyone can wear. In most cases, they guarantee neither licensing nor specific training. You must quiz each of these professionals closely, because their business cards rarely reveal what they actually do.

A good financial advisor is hard to find, but a good financial advisor will take the burden of planning your finances off your shoulders. You will still have to stay in touch with your money, your expenses, and your investments, and you will still have to take responsible actions. But, you will no longer be alone, and you will have far more mental energy to devote to your career, your family, and your joys in life.

MOVING TOWARD FINANCIAL HEALTH

No single book could ever teach you to be a good doctor. And in this book, I will not teach you how to be your own financial advisor. Not only would that take years of training, but the market, the laws, and the strategies change so often that no one could ever do these jobs well by doing them part time.

Instead, I will educate you about the pillars, strategies, and pitfalls of wealth management, so you can select and use a financial advisor or wealth manager wisely.

Together, you can then work toward your greatest possible financial health.

CHAPTER ONE

Macro Challenges

If you practice medicine in the United States, I don't need to tell you that a tsunami of change has hit your profession. But these changes are caused by more than politics.

Just as tsunamis are driven by major earthquakes beneath the sea, the changes in US health care are driven by a powerful underlying crisis: Our country spends a whopping 20 percent of our gross domestic product (GDP) on health care, but residents of the United States have a shorter life expectancy and greater prevalence of chronic conditions than do people in other advanced nations. Japan spends only about 7 percent of its GDP on health care, but the overall health of its population is better.

That means we're doing something massively wrong.

In addition, the basic health-care entitlement programs in the United States are facing fiscal crises at the same time as our overall population is becoming progressively older. As of this writing, the Medicare trust fund is heading for bankruptcy in about fifteen years. Medicaid has an uncertain political future.

Politicians on both the left and the right have been scrambling to remake the system. They may disagree on the answers, but they do ask the same question: *How do we improve health-care delivery while spending less?*

No one likes change, and doctors are no exception. Indeed, many physicians remain nostalgic for the "good old days" of health care—when doctors made the rules, money was thrown around with few controls, and insurance companies had far less power.

But those days are over.

We don't know the future economics of health care, but we do know that regardless of who comes to power, we will see reform, and that reform will include cuts in payments to physicians. You will be required to take more risk. You will be asked to deliver better and more efficient services. You will be asked to work longer hours with more monitoring and regulations.

That said, I am confident that doctoring will remain a lucrative profession. The rising demand for care and the sheer size of the health-care economy will guarantee it. The United States spends about $3.8 *trillion* on health care each year. If the US health-care industry were a country, it would be the fifth largest economy in the world, right behind Germany and ahead of the United Kingdom. When you are an essential part of 20 percent of the GDP in the wealthiest country on earth and a leading citizen of the fifth largest economic unit ever created, you are going to make money.

Keeping that money is another matter altogether.

You will keep your money only if you pay attention to the direction of the coming storms—only if you solidify your financial defenses and prepare for any change on the horizon.

A LITTLE HISTORY

To understand how we got to the present economic crisis for American physicians, it's worth looking back.

Until a few decades ago, the fiscal relationship between doctor and patient was straightforward. It was called, simply, "billed charge." A patient went to see a doctor, the doctor sent a bill, and the patient paid the doctor.

If the patient could not pay the bill, the doctor would not see them anymore. As a result, a lot of people, especially older people, simply could not afford medical care. They died younger, and they died in poor health.

In those days, *some* people carried medical insurance but not the general population.

A lot of dentistry still functions on the billed charge model, and dentists continue to work in much the same way as doctors worked in my grandfather's time. Although some people carry dental insurance, many dentists still set their own rates and charge their patients directly. They also work under much lighter regulation than doctors.

In the old days, doctors and patients would sometimes bargain directly over the price of care. A patient would either pay full price or decide to go elsewhere. In general, this worked beautifully for doctors, even if patients were often forced to live without care.

One of my clients is a retired Ob-Gyn who practiced in New York. He told me that within a few years of starting his practice in the 1960s, he was netting $3 million a year. Today, a typical Ob-Gyn makes about a tenth of that. Now, $300,000 to $500,000 a year is still very good money, but it's not the *crazy money* made in those days.

How could this Ob-Gyn have made so much? People wanted to give birth safely to a child, so they were willing to pay whatever he asked. No insurance company told him what he could bill, and no government agency was watching.

The doctor could *bill and bill and bill* without regulation.

ENTER MEDICARE AND MEDICAID

In 1965, President Lyndon Johnson drove through the creation of Medicare to give health insurance to everyone sixty-five and older, regardless of their income or health situation. Medicaid was part of the same legislation; it gave aid to the poor at any age.

The typical life expectancy in the 1960s was only about 69.7 years. When the Medicare Act went through, Congress expected people to die before they collected many years of benefits. If you retired at sixty-five, the government thought it would have to cover you for only about five years. The whole program seemed not too costly.

As people began living longer, however, a huge percentage of the population began to rely on Medicare. The typical American life expectancy is now seventy-eight—an enormous increase from the inception of the program.

As Medicare became the biggest health insurance program in the nation, it began to reshape the fundamental fiscal relationship between doctor and patient. Little by little, doctors no longer billed patients directly. They billed Medicare or Medicaid, and these programs would not accept the doctors' full price for many procedures. The doctor would bill $1,000. Medicare would say, "No, I'm going to pay you $200."

When doctors negotiated with patients, all the power was in the hands of the doctor. Now, doctors had to negotiate with the government, and the government had much more power to set prices than any mere patient negotiating his or her own rate.

Private insurance companies grew in power in parallel to Medicare and Medicaid, and they followed the same model of determining pricing for physicians. Indeed, whatever prices the government set, the private insurance market usually followed their lead.

For a while, many physicians continued to operate under the old system in their private practices, but gradually, the government and private insurance companies took over the bulk of *all* health-care finance. Today, the majority of doctors accept both Medicare payment regulations and the complex payment rules set by leading private insurance companies.

In our time, only a very few, highly successful doctors can avoid the insurance system and set their own pricing directly with patients as "concierge doctors."

THE MEDICAL MARKET BOOM

Importantly, because of Medicare, Medicaid, and private insurance, many more people could afford health care. As a result, the nation saw an enormous boom in the medical market—more appointments, more tests, and more of everything.

Doctors may not have been able to charge whatever they wanted for a patient's visit, but they got many more visits, so doctoring remained a high-income profession.

Of course, the boom changed much more than the financials in the doctor-patient relationship. In the old days, a doctor might spend a whole hour, even two, with a patient. They'd get to know the patient, establish a personal relationship, and they would bill for the privilege. But now, because insurance reimburses only each visit rather than each minute spent with a patient, doctors try to cram as many patients as they can into a single hour.

Medicare might pay, say, $56 per visit. But, if doctors could spend just six minutes with each patient, they could bill

Medicare for ten visits in one hour and earn $560 an hour. Accidentally exceed that six minutes per visit, and revenues went way down.

The overall insurance model created an additional *adverse incentive* for both doctor and patient. If the patient remained sick, he or she would visit more times. The patient wouldn't mind visiting again and again, because their policy paid for unlimited visits.

In the old days, under direct charge, a patient would think hard before every expensive visit to a doctor. And if treatments did not seem to be going well, it was easier to change doctors, because the patient did not need to stay within the same network. Although doctors had much greater power, this did offer some minor bargaining clout to the patient, as well as a higher incentive for the doctor to do a good job.

Medicare worked well for a few decades before it began to run out of money. Estimates say the average retiree will use about three times as much Medicare health-care money as he or she put into the system. And indeed, money pours out of the Medicare fund at about three times the rate as the money pouring in.

At some point, everyone realized that the US health-care model had become unsustainable.

ENTER OBAMACARE

Beginning in 2008, the Obama administration tried to deal with the overall crisis with the partisan ACA. In 2015 came the bipartisan Medicare Access and CHIP Reauthorization Act (MACRA), CHIP standing for Children's Health Insurance Program.

The goals of the ACA were admirable: increase access to affordable health care by expanding insurance coverage. Reduce the growth of health-care spending. Improve the efficiencies of health-care deliveries.

Unfortunately, much of the burden of achieving these goals fell on the shoulders of physicians. Obamacare significantly reduced the number of uninsured individuals and expanded the patient pool for physicians. Like the introduction of Medicare and Medicaid, it flooded the system; these new patients tended to be poorer and sicker, because they had not had insurance before Obamacare, and their treatments might have been delayed.

The greater number of patients might still have benefited physicians overall, except that among its many provisions and strategies, the ACA introduced the "value-based," or result-based, reimbursement model. Under the current provisions, of which very little is discussed in the media, physicians have to prove the value of their treatments.

As all doctors who accept Medicare know, you may no longer automatically receive payment when you submit a bill to the government. Medicare wants to see the results of your treatments. If the results fall below average, they will penalize you with a reduced payment, and if your results are above average, you will receive a bonus. Indeed, if your results are very good—if your patients see you just once and get healthy—you will get a big bonus.

In other words, value-based reimbursement attempts to correlate the number of visits with the outcome of visits. If a patient goes back to you after a week for the same procedure, it's an indication that your first procedure produced no positive result, so you will get reimbursed only once instead of twice.

If executed properly, this system would indeed encourage doctors to work harder on keeping their patients healthy, instead of encouraging as many return visits as possible. Medicare would also benefit. By attempting to remove the adverse incentive, the framers of the ACA hoped to preserve the Medicare trust fund, or at least extend its life a few more years. And indeed, as of this writing, the *increase* in Medicare costs has been reduced, and the *speed* in the overall increase in health-care costs has been reduced quite substantially.

Meanwhile, however, *overall costs* continue to rise, and it has become clear that the ACA will not solve the bigger problem or save the Medicare trust fund. Why? The fundamentals have not changed. People live longer. Researchers keep inventing more and more expensive procedures to prolong life. More people use these expensive procedures. Net result: a poor financial prognosis for the system.

VALUE-BASED REIMBURSEMENT HERE TO STAY?

The MACRA bill of 2015 included lots of complexity, but one of its most important goals was to streamline the value-based reimbursement system that had been worked out in the ACA. Importantly, MACRA passed as a bipartisan bill, which means that whatever reforms the Republicans bring in the next few years, *value-based reimbursement is probably here to stay*.

Billed charges have largely disappeared; even pure fee-for-service (FFS) is on its way out. In their place will inevitably come various value-based reimbursement systems, such as the Merit-Based Incentive Payment System (MIPS) and alternative payment models (APMs). If MIPS is fully implemented as planned in 2022, physicians could get incentive and bonus adjustments of up to 37 percent of payments or penalties of up to 9 percent of payments—as the Centers for Medicare and Medicaid Services (CMS) attempt to keep the incentives and penalties budget-neutral. Suffice it to say, a good chunk of physician incomes will be at risk.

Being a physician was never a low-stress job. But in the new world introduced by Medicare and other insurance, doctors went beyond their daily responsibilities for life and death to a high-wire financial game in which they had to choose how much time to spend with each patient and which insurance plans to accept.

Under the ACA, this stress hit new heights. Not only did physicians have to worry about value-based reimbursement, but the ACA upped the level of charting and coding for every procedure in an attempt to micromanage the medical process.

Why? Because value and results' monitoring requires *a lot* of data.

The Business of Charting and Coding

Patients showed up poorer, sicker, and in bigger numbers. But under the ACA, doctors had to do more than increase their healing work. They had to increase their personal administrative overhead exponentially, along with a geometric expansion of the emotional EMR overwhelm that I mentioned in the introduction.

Every practicing physician today knows about the stress of

the increasing number and granularity of treatment codes. You must learn literally tens of thousands of different codes, and the system has become extraordinarily complicated.

Often, similar treatments can be coded differently for insurance purposes with vastly different reimbursements. As a result, coding itself has become a business, with its own risks and rewards.

Every doctor understands this unfortunate truth. Let me give you an example from a patient's point of view.

Good Coding Can Pay More Than Good Medicine

When my child was born, the doctor said the shape of his ear did not look quite right. So the doctor decided to put a device, a kind of small plastic box, on my baby's ear to make it grow into a better shape. But when he was attaching the box to the ear—a procedure that took about ten minutes—the doctor used a razor to shave a few hairs behind the ear that would have interfered.

No big deal? Wrong. When my wife looked at the bill from the insurance company, she saw that the procedure was coded as "surgery," and the charge was $2,000 for those ten minutes.

How could this be surgery? Well, the doctor had used a

blade to cut those hairs, had he not? The insurance company could not argue and didn't seem to care. To them, it was just a cost of doing business. My wife was livid and so was I. We were sure this doctor was abusing the system. We were also certain the system was broken.

Now, I'm sure many honest doctors don't try to make money through cagey coding. Most doctors work long hours just trying to understand the system and ensuring they're not making simple coding errors that will bring the wrath of Medicare or an insurance company lawyer down onto their backs.

Indeed, as we discussed earlier, the increased burden of charting has alone resulted in an epidemic of physician burnout and a significant increase in the number of physician suicides.

AFTER THE ACA

As of this writing, it's too early to say what will happen to key provisions of the ACA under the new Republican administration and Congress. It's likely that the ACA exchanges will eventually collapse, and we may see many more uninsured Americans, but it may take years to repeal the ACA altogether, with or without a replacement.

However, as noted earlier, the bipartisan passage of MACRA

probably means the fundamental idea of value-based reimbursement will retain Republican support and will survive the collapse of the ACA. Because value-based reimbursement is among the most stressful changes facing physicians, we can be pretty sure that physician stress will not be reduced.

And we can be entirely certain that uncertainty will persist.

Although physicians cannot hope to take full political control of the health-care debate, they should get involved and stay involved in advocacy through physician political action committees (PACs).

You can have an important voice in new policies, even if you may not have the most powerful voice. No one doubts that the pharmaceutical companies and insurance companies will continue to have greater clout than doctors, who are dispersed into many different kinds of organizations and small businesses. Insurance and Big Pharma have deeper pockets, more strings to pull, and better lobbyists than doctors could ever dream of sending into the battle.

THE RISE OF MEDICAL CORPORATIONS

One of the most important macro changes impacting physicians is the accelerating demise of the private practice.

With the rise of *Big Insurance* came the rise of big medical corporations—partly due to the heavy administrative burden of modern health care, partly due to the need for clout to push back against insurance companies, and partly due to the stress and burnout of physicians trying to make it in private practice under new regulations.

You can draw a direct parallel to the way in which mom-and-pop shops gave way to the Walmart's of the world, the way independent bookstores fell to big chains, and the way franchise restaurant chains took over all the major freeway intersections in America. The "retail" business of health care seems to be headed in the same direction as retail in general.

All across the country, we see older doctors retiring earlier from their practices, and younger docs choosing to work in big medical corporations, institutions, and hospitals. This new generation wants to do their medical work *and then go home*. Instead of hanging out a shingle, younger docs are increasingly looking to careers treating patients in a Kaiser or other large-scale system, doing research in facilities such as the National Institutes of Health, or working in medically oriented Silicon Valley start-ups.

Of private practice, younger docs often say, "I just don't want the hassle."

Certainly, those who do choose to go into private practice must assemble more outside professional help than ever before. Private physicians need to identify a team that includes a good certified public accountant (CPA), a practice consultant, an insurance expert, and an attorney. If you go into private practice, don't go it alone.

PROTECTING YOURSELF FROM THE MACRO

Let me end this brief discussion of macro challenges with the simple observation that you cannot ultimately control the macro environment in which you practice; you can control only your own response to that environment. The waves of the tsunami are not going to subside anytime soon. No political party will come to rescue your finances. And we will never return to the "good old days."

You must build a solid financial structure that will survive the biggest waves—a house to withstand any storms that might blow your way.

In the next chapter, we will move from the macro to the micro and look at the unique personal financial challenges confronting every physician. In Chapter 3, I will tell you a few important stories about physicians who came to me for help after falling victim to these challenges. Then, we will begin to construct your new financial home.

CHAPTER TWO

Personal Challenges

Do doctors still make good money?

In 2016, the median US household income was just over
$51,000. Meanwhile, the median income for the lowest-
earning medical specialty, pediatrician, was over $200,000.
That's four times the median US household income. Ortho-
pedists earned a median of $443,000, with cardiologists a
close second, at $410,000.

Here's a 2016 snapshot of median physician incomes, by
specialty. Despite all the social and political challenges we
discussed in the preceding chapter, the average American
would still find this chart pretty impressive:

How Much Do Physicians Earn Overall?

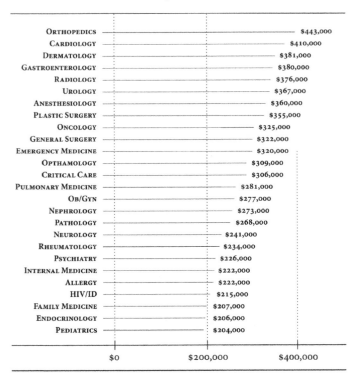

ORTHOPEDICS		$443,000
CARDIOLOGY		$410,000
DERMATOLOGY		$381,000
GASTROENTEROLOGY		$380,000
RADIOLOGY		$376,000
UROLOGY		$367,000
ANESTHESIOLOGY		$360,000
PLASTIC SURGERY		$355,000
ONCOLOGY		$325,000
GENERAL SURGERY		$322,000
EMERGENCY MEDICINE		$320,000
OPTHAMOLOGY		$309,000
CRITICAL CARE		$306,000
PULMONARY MEDICINE		$281,000
OB/GYN		$277,000
NEPHROLOGY		$273,000
PATHOLOGY		$268,000
NEUROLOGY		$241,000
RHEUMATOLOGY		$234,000
PSYCHIATRY		$226,000
INTERNAL MEDICINE		$222,000
ALLERGY		$222,000
HIV/ID		$215,000
FAMILY MEDICINE		$207,000
ENDOCRINOLOGY		$206,000
PEDIATRICS		$204,000

$0 $200,000 $400,000

Credit: Medscape

Why, then, do so few physicians accumulate substantial wealth over the course of their careers? In the introduction, we looked at some docs who were ten or more years into highly successful careers but had few assets to show for it.

In this chapter, we'll see why such tales are sadly common.

THE TOP SIX HURDLES

After talking to hundreds of doctors and working with many dozens in my financial advisory, I have come to see the same patterns repeat themselves. Now, when I sit down with a new physician client, I break out their personal challenges into six very common hurdles.

1. YOU DON'T KNOW WHAT YOU ARE DOING

I'm sorry, but most physicians just don't know much about wealth management. Medical schools don't teach personal finance, and there's no rotation into a wealth management firm during residency.

I also find that medicine has a different fiscal orientation from almost any other profession on earth; it exists in a financial universe of its own. Handling your own wealth takes an important mental shift from "saving lives at any cost" and "prescribing drugs without knowing their price tag" to "living within a budget" and "investing for the future."

Many doctors can't seem to make that shift, to think in long-term dollars and sense—pun intended. In my experience, only about 5 percent of physicians have the knowledge they need to handle their own wealth.

2. YOU GET A LATE START, CARRYING HUGE STUDENT DEBT

In the introduction, I discussed my young friend Rajesh, who was coming out of fifteen years of higher education at the age of thirty-five with nothing in the bank and $300,000 debt in student loans. For more than twelve years, since the age of twenty-two, when most educated people begin earning money and building a financial base, he had been in classrooms and labs, as well as working hospital shifts with a token income.

Rajesh hardly represents an unusual case. Indeed, he managed to start practicing before many of his peers, who did not get their licenses until their late thirties. And plenty of his fellow classmates started with the additional burden of a family to support, even a mortgage to pay. Nearly every one of them had huge student debts hanging over their heads, with many of those debts much higher than his $300,000.

Doctors may earn good money, but they have less time to earn and less time to invest those earnings. This represents a challenge that all too many ignore.

3. YOUR LIFESTYLE EXPECTATIONS ARE HIGH

Doctors face enormous social pressure to live in a big house in a nice neighborhood, drive a luxury car, own a vacation home, eat in fancy restaurants, and send their kids to private schools. They see their colleagues sporting this lifestyle, and they may feel that their spouse "married a doctor," expecting nothing less.

Adding to this pressure is the PMF syndrome, the pent-up monetary frustration that I diagnosed in the case of Rajesh. After a third of a lifetime spent looking longingly out the windows of schools and hospital towers, doctors are ready to enjoy themselves, and they don't want to hear anyone telling them to delay gratification right into middle age.

As in the case of Doc Edwards, come middle age, the pressure to show the fruit of all that labor becomes especially intense. Despite a healthy income, however, most doctors find it tough to both live like a highflier *and* accumulate a high-class portfolio.

4. YOU DON'T HAVE ENOUGH TIME AND ENERGY FOR YOUR MONEY

Medicine makes extreme mental, even physical, demands. And in today's environment, you have to do much more than see patients; you have to spend a lot of your working day staring at a computer to do enervating administrative and regulatory chores.

By the time you get home, you find it tough to get back in front of a screen and figure out your personal finances— really tough. You also don't have time to read books on finance or take classes.

5. YOU ATTRACT SCAMMERS AND DUBIOUS INVESTMENT SCHEMES

Unscrupulous brokers, hedge fund managers, real estate aggregators, insurance fund salespeople, and get-rich-quick scammers of all stripes love to target doctors. They know you have a high income, they know you have acquired significant assets without a proper education in financial issues, and they know you don't have time to look deeply into their "investments."

Worthless schemes can come from criminals, from big-name investment houses, or from friends and relatives. Regardless of the origin, badly conceived investments suck the wealth right out of smart, highly educated professionals who would never be fooled by a dubious lab result or a lame previous diagnosis. As you will see in Chapter 3, the toll can be catastrophic.

6. YOU DON'T SEE THE VALUE IN FINANCIAL ADVISORS

I discussed this issue at some length in the introduction,

and I rank distrust of advisors right up there among the most significant issues facing physicians.

It's true that the quality of financial advisors varies wildly, but the services of an expert are as essential to wealth management as they are to health management. Later, I will offer an extended discussion of how to choose a qualified financial advisor and use them wisely. But here's a hint: *It begins with separating advisors from salespeople.*

CLEAR AND PRESENT DANGER

They don't teach you how to cope with these six vital personal challenges in medical school. But in the next chapter, we will see how they represent a real and present danger to your health, happiness, and career.

CHAPTER THREE

Cautionary Tales

The six hurdles presented in Chapter 2 prevent the majority of physicians from accumulating substantial wealth and living the lives they deserve. That's because any single hurdle can trip up even the most successful doctor and lead to devastating financial mistakes.

Now I want to open up my files and look at some case histories. All these stories are true, but of course, the names have been changed. Each is a cautionary tale, and I think the lessons are pretty clear.

CANCER IN THE PORTFOLIO

Dr. Anderson has become a multimillionaire physician with sizable investments, but he has never had much time to choose them wisely. Until recently, he depended on a storied Wall Street brokerage. This brokerage paid their senior executives $4 billion in the same year the firm needed a federal bailout. During that famous year, three of Dr. Anderson's accounts lost a great deal of money. The personal hurdle he faced? Not the big market crash but big-name market *scammers*.

DOUBLE-DEALING IN TREASURIES

One of Dr. Anderson's investments was a US Treasury account, through which his big-name money manager purchased Treasury bills and bonds on his behalf. The year 2008 might have been bad for stocks, but it was a great year for all US Treasury securities.

The stock turmoil caused investors to flock to Treasuries, driving prices up between 3 percent and 13 percent. Dr. Anderson's Treasury account, however, lost 3 percent.

What could cause a discrepancy like this? Well, his "full-service" brokerage also worked as a primary dealer in the Treasury market. They bought securities and *resold them* to their customers at a huge markup, which effectively wiped out all client profits and even put some clients into the negative.

The brokerage made money; Dr. Anderson did not—hence,

the big bonuses to senior executives at the storied Wall Street firm.

CHURNING STOCKS

In that same year of 2008, the Standard & Poor's (S&P) 500 Index lost 38 percent. However, Dr. Anderson's stock account lost 62 percent. How could that happen? Well, the brokerage performed frequent trades, including extremely high volumes of buys and sells of largely S&P 500 stocks in small lots. His year-end statement had no less than 377 pages of transaction records. The sheer volume of trade fees and taxes was devastating to him. Once again, of course, the brokerage did just fine.

HEDGE FUND ROULETTE

Many Wall Street financial firms like to tell their wealthy clients that they can put their money in investments not available to the general public. Sure enough, Dr. Anderson's broker put nearly 40 percent of his money into a hedge fund.

The good news? To this day, the hedge fund reports that it's "making money." The bad news? These results are not audited or even calculated by a third party.

At last check, the fund was headquartered in Paris, and the

Securities and Exchange Commission (SEC) had no record of either the fund or its managers. Could this be another Bernie Madoff-style scam? We still can't be sure.

THE LESSON OF DR. ANDERSON

What can we learn from this unfortunate physician? *Never hire a Wall Street broker to be your financial advisor. They don't work for you; they work for themselves.*

EXORBITANT HIDDEN COSTS

Dr. Zuck was a middle-class primary care physician. He was not as wealthy as Dr. Anderson, so he was harder to rip off through something like a hedge fund. All of his investments were plain-vanilla mutual funds arranged by another major national brokerage through his financial advisor.

Sounds safe? Well, maybe not.

When we look closely at each of these mutual funds, we will find that they all featured enormous hidden costs. Here's a breakdown for one year, with some of the *exorbitant* numbers highlighted in darker shading. Merely *bad* numbers are shaded more lightly.

Symbol	Expense	Load	Turnover
CAIBX	0.59%	5.75%	63%
CAPCX	1.66%	1%	89%
FEVCX	1.90%	1%	15%
MIQBX	1.30%	5.25%	29%
OIBIX	0.57%	None	111%
WAFMX	2.25%	None	34%
WFPAX	1.24%	5.75%	58%

Doctors can read medical charts with precision, but unlike most investors, they rarely learn how to read fund charts, and they even more rarely research the comparisons to other kinds of investments. What most middle-class investors consider "safe" can actually be a rip-off.

READING THE CHART

Mutual funds come with three primary hidden costs. When brokers, masquerading as financial advisors, sell you such funds, they are under no obligation to disclose these costs to you. And remember again that about 93 percent of "financial advisors" are actually brokers.

Expense ratio shows the percentage of your assets that you pay in annual fees to the fund managers. These fees are yearly and recurring—therefore, becoming extraordinarily expensive over time.

The best mutual funds are usually index funds or asset-class funds offering an expense ratio of around 0.1 percent. The lowest-cost index fund has an expense ratio of only 0.03 percent. When you compare those kinds of rates, *which may feature nearly identical stock portfolios* to the mutual funds in Dr. Zuck's "safe" investment, you can see he was paying his managers ten to sixty times more than necessary—every single year.

Why does this happen? Funds with high expense ratios are generally funds that cannot sell themselves. Hence, they need to give "financial advisors" (in this case, actual brokers) huge kickbacks to add them to their clients' portfolios. A high expense ratio simply finances the kickback to your broker. It's that simple.

Load represents the initial commission paid to the "financial advisor" (once again, actually your broker) for directing a client's money into the fund. You should never pay any load at all, because you can find so many top-notch no-load funds out there. If you pay your financial advisor a fee, and he or she collects a load on top of that, it's plain-vanilla double-dipping. Unfortunately, double-dipping is common when you hire a broker as a financial advisor.

Turnover is the most hidden of hidden costs. It shows how often the fund churns itself with buy and sell orders. The higher the churn rate, the higher the internal fund transaction costs and tax costs to investors. One good estimate translates a 100 percent turnover rate into 1.2 percent in return drag, meaning *money lost*. The best funds have a turnover rate of only 5 percent, not the staggeringly high churns shown in Dr. Zuck's portfolio.

THE LESSON OF DR. ZUCK

Hidden costs can impoverish you. Let the buyer beware.

TOO MUCH HOUSE

I know I keep mentioning houses, but what can I say? Doctors like big houses.

Dr. and Mrs. Shah came to the United States from South Asia. They dreamed a big American dream, a dream so big they needed a stunningly big house in an undeniably fancy neighborhood to contain it.

In 1989, they bought a sixteen-thousand-square-foot mansion outside an East Coast city. It had ten bedrooms, nine bathrooms, an indoor swimming pool, and an outdoor tennis court. They spent $2.5 million to purchase this house and another $500,000 to renovate it.

Fast-forward to 2017. Dr. and Mrs. Shah have hit their seventies, but they have not yet paid off their mortgage. Their monthly payment still runs at nearly $10,000. On top of that, property tax and maintenance costs on the house, grounds, pool, and so on run a staggering $150,000 a year. In other words, these good people spend $270,000 every single year on this mansion.

Ironically, Dr. and Mrs. Shah do not swim, they do not play tennis, and they cannot possibly be using all ten bedrooms and nine bathrooms.

If you think this couple has recouped their investment through property appreciation over nearly three decades, you're wrong. As of now, the property is worth only $2 million for a variety of local real estate reasons. The value has declined, even though I calculate that Dr. Shah has sunk more than $7 million into this house if you include initial purchase, renovation, and annual expenses.

Despite the incredible yearly cost, Dr. Shah is reluctant to sell out at such a huge loss. But because he desired, and still desires, the facade of living large, he sadly could not retire when he turned seventy. The math is simple. His retirement savings stand at $2 million, which might be good enough for many folks to make a comfortable retirement. But in his case, every penny of that money would be eaten up by the mansion in a mere seven years. Unless he gives up the facade, he cannot afford to stop working.

THE LESSON OF DR. SHAH

Do not become a slave to your house.

"GOING BARE"

Dr. Marcus, a well-known Ob-Gyn, practiced in a large metropolitan area for more than twenty-five years. He built a highly successful practice, and he did not make any of the financial mistakes of Drs. Anderson, Zuck, or Shah. During his career, he accumulated a sizable net worth by living within his means, saving a significant portion of his income, and making some shrewd investments.

During the last five years of his practice, however, Dr. Marcus was sued three times. Most physicians and lawyers would refer to these lawsuits as "nuisance suits." Nonetheless, these nuisances proved expensive for his malpractice insurer to defend.

In each instance, even though Dr. Marcus's counsel believed his client had a strong defense, which would have prevailed at trial, the insurance company's counsel elected to settle for what it believed to be nominal sums ranging from $25,000 to $40,000.

As a consequence, insurance companies now considered Dr. Marcus a high risk. By the end of the third case, Dr. Marcus's annual malpractice premium had more than tripled, to almost half of his annual salary.

Rather than continue to pay this exorbitant fee, Dr. Marcus elected to "go bare," without any malpractice insurance at all. It was a terrible mistake.

A short time later, he was sued again, because one of his patients gave birth to a severely handicapped baby. This was, of course, more than a nuisance suit. Most experts agreed that Dr. Marcus conducted himself in an appropriate manner during the birth of this baby and treatment of his patient. They said he lost the case only because the jury felt tremendous compassion for the plaintiff's situation and believed that *someone should pay*. Apparently a "wealthy physician" was the best candidate.

The judgment was in the millions, and Dr. Marcus lost literally all the assets he had saved through an entire career of work. Perhaps the jury would be pleased to learn he was wealthy no more.

THE LESSON OF DR. MARCUS

Never, ever leave your assets unprotected.

PLAYING AT UNRELATED BUSINESSES

Dr. Gold works as a partner in an emergency medical practice that nets him a substantial $1 million annual income. Despite this success, when he approached me for advice, I was shocked to discover he had only about $100,000 in savings. If he experienced his own emergency, those savings would be enough to cover his personal expenses for only about two months.

Without any doubt, this ER doc lived an extravagant lifestyle that ate up plenty of his income. But the big problem was his real estate investments.

In 2007, at the persistent urging of a high school buddy, Dr. Gold had purchased three office buildings. His buddy had convinced him that because these buildings were in a less desirable neighborhood "ready to pop," they were supposedly way underpriced and certain to double in value over the ensuing three years.

Unfortunately, Dr. Gold bought these buildings just before the commercial real estate market tanked in the financial crisis of 2008. Nine years later, none of the three has yet to recover even its original value.

Meanwhile, the upkeep and rental of his commercial properties have become serious financial and emotional burdens for Dr. Gold—not to mention a daily distraction from his practice. Despite all the money he has spent over the years, his buildings have fallen into disrepair, and the tenants have been leaving in droves. Lately, the good doctor has been spending a lot of his time on the phone begging tenants to stay.

None of this, of course, has anything to do with the business Dr. Gold knows well—medicine. Although he continues to make a huge profit from his practice, it's barely enough to cover the red ink in his real estate business. Worse yet, as of this writing, he holds on to the hope that his buildings' value may still, someday, double.

THE LESSON OF DR. GOLD

Do what you are good at doing. Stop doing what you are not good at doing.

PRIVATE INVESTMENTS WITH A RELATIVE

Not just the buddies but also the close relatives of doctors often try to draw them into dubious investment schemes.

Dr. Morris practices as a podiatrist with a respectable

income. He lives a relatively frugal life in Los Angeles. Early in his career, he accumulated about $1 million in savings. Unfortunately, he had no idea how to invest that money wisely.

One day, a relative of Dr. Morris approached him about investing in an online video game start-up backed by a well-known entertainment celebrity. It was an exciting, late-night conversation, and he had to promise absolute secrecy. You won't be surprised to learn that Dr. Morris knew nothing about the video game industry, Hollywood stars, or entertainment, in general. So, he thought, *What could possibly go wrong with a venture vouched for by a trusted relative and backed by a famous Hollywood star?*

The good doctor put half a million dollars into the venture, hoping to one day strike it big and turn that $500,000 into $1 billion, just like Peter Thiel did with his investment in Facebook. Within a few weeks, however, the Hollywood star (who had lent only his fame but had invested no actual capital) backed out of the project. The CEO of the start-up turned out to have another company of his own, and the investors learned of dubious financial transactions between the new start-up and this other concern.

Along with the other shareholders, Dr. Morris filed a lawsuit and became deeply embroiled in the resulting cost and hassle. The good news? The shareholders won, and they gained full control of the online game start-up company. The bad news? Not one of them had the faintest idea how to run an online game start-up. And of course, they got none of their money back.

"I haven't learned much about gaming," the podiatrist told me. "But I learned quite a lot about the securities laws." I was reminded of a quote from Warren Buffet: "When a man with money does business with a man with experience, the man with experience will end up with the money, and the man with money will end up with experience."

THE LESSON OF DR. MORRIS

Stay away from private investments, even with relatives—maybe especially with relatives.

YOUR "FRIEND," THE INSURANCE AGENT

Dr. Chang arrived on our shores as an immigrant from Taiwan and began serving the local Chinese immigrant community. His wife works in the home. They married young, and at sixty, they have two grown sons and three fine grandchildren.

Like many other immigrants from less developed countries,

Dr. Chang finds himself befuddled by the array of financial products available in the United States, and he distrusts American financial professionals. When it comes to money matters, he relies only on his inner circle.

One woman in this inner circle acts as an insurance agent for a big life insurance company. She persuaded the doctor to buy $2 million worth of "permanent life insurance" for himself and his wife, and $1 million each for his two children and three young grandchildren. This agent convinced him that "life insurance is the best gift you can give your loved ones."

The premiums would be $70,000 per year for the rest of his life, nearly one-sixth of his pretax income.

After he signed the documents, Dr. Chang realized he could not actually keep paying $70,000 a year for this policy, and he began to have buyer's regret.

When he approached me about extricating himself from this situation, I asked, "How on earth did this woman persuade you to buy all this life insurance? The purpose of life insurance is to insure against the financial risk of someone dying prematurely—not to 'give a gift' to anyone."

Indeed, Dr. Chang's children were fully grown and supporting themselves admirably. His grandchildren were still young, but they were not his responsibility; they were the responsibility of his sons and daughters-in-law.

But Dr. Chang bought insurance on his own life and on the lives of his sons; and incredibly, this "friend" had even persuaded the good doctor to insure the lives of his grandchildren—the youngest a baby. The grandchildren had no financial responsibility for anyone, so there was no possible argument for insuring against their premature deaths.

How had this happened? How had he made this staggering financial decision?

Well, when Dr. Chang and his wife came to America, they found they deeply missed the cuisine from their home country, especially good Chinese dumplings. They would look far and wide to find really authentic dumplings.

One Sunday morning, the friendly insurance agent brought over some dumplings her mother had made. "When my mom made these, I immediately thought of you two. I'm sure you will enjoy her dumplings."

The dumplings were very good—the real deal. And for a time, every single Sunday, the agent brought over more fresh dumplings her mother had made. It became a special time for the three friends to get together.

One Sunday, when their friendship had deepened, and as they were sitting around the kitchen table eating these amazing dumplings, the remarkable friend brought out all the paperwork from the New York insurance company, saying, "Here is a fantastic investment, not just for you but also for your grandchildren. I really believe in this, and I think you should buy these policies right away."

Before they realized exactly what the policies entailed or the size of their commitment, Dr. Chang and his wife signed.

I asked them, "After you signed the papers and bought the insurance, did the agent still come back to serve you her mother's dumplings every Sunday morning?"

"Well, no," answered Dr. Chang and his wife. After they signed, both the agent and the dumplings became scarce. In fact, the Changs now had a hard time getting her on the phone.

No doubt, this agent is now busy bringing her mother's dumplings to other rich Chinese Americans.

As we will see in the next chapter, permanent life insurance usually represents a very bad investment, and it is very different from term life insurance. Physicians with young families are wise to obtain some term life insurance for about twenty years, until their children are old enough to work for themselves and before accumulating sufficient assets and investments to support a nonworking spouse in case of a tragedy. After that, any kind of life insurance rarely makes sense.

The agent had endangered Dr. Chang's financial stability and his hopes for retirement, while helping ensure her own.

THE LESSON OF DR. CHANG

An insurance agent is not your *agent.*

SERIOUS CHARITY TAKES LONG-TERM PLANNING

Dr. Farooq also made his way to the United States to practice medicine. He and his wife came from a war-torn Middle Eastern country, and here they prospered. Dr. Farooq founded five urgent-care clinics—making good money when he owned them and good money when he sold them off. Now, he's retired.

Throughout her husband's medical career, Mrs. Farooq had been a highly supportive spouse and had made many personal sacrifices. Dr. Farooq now feels the time has come to support her in her own pursuits, which include an ambitious charity.

Mrs. Farooq has a deep commitment to helping girls in her home country, and for decades, she has nursed the dream of starting a girls' school offering a Western-style education. Now that her husband has retired, she feels empowered to take action.

The couple estimate they will need $100,000 in capital just to get the project off the ground, with much more needed later on. They are so committed to this cause that they're willing to spend their retirement funds to make it happen.

But here's the problem. Now that Dr. Farooq no longer works, they have no income against which to write off these expenses. They will receive little tax benefit from their charitable effort, making it twice as expensive for them.

Mrs. Farooq had her idea for a girls' school long ago. If the couple had worked with a financial advisor and started a donor-advised fund (see Chapter 4) while the doctor was still bringing in a substantial amount of money, they could have written off *all* the charitable expenses against Dr. Farooq's significant income—*before those expenses occurred.*

Unfortunately, the couple never sought advice or took this action, so now, whatever they spend will have to come directly out of their own funds, impacting their retirement and limiting the good they will do.

THE LESSON OF DR. FAROOQ

Advance charitable planning saves taxes and maximizes your impact.

SUCCESS REQUIRES A SUCCESSION PLAN

Dr. Williams was a dedicated gastroenterologist. Since he had started practicing twenty-three years ago, he regularly worked ten-hour days, six days a week. Thanks to these efforts, he had built a huge patient panel of well over four thousand individuals.

If he had decided to sell this thriving practice, it could easily have fetched more than $500,000. But at middle age, Dr. Williams hadn't given much thought to business succession planning. It sat on his to-do list but was always pushed back to make room for more urgent matters. After all, he was in good health, and he foresaw many more working years ahead.

Then, a year ago, Dr. Williams was diagnosed with an aggressive lymphoma. Within months, he died of the disease.

Unfortunately, he did not go with peace of mind. On his deathbed, Dr. Williams was still frantically calling other doctors in the area and pleading with them to take his patients. During his last days, a large number of his patients still did not have a new physician, and he felt guilty about it. Even worse, he realized he was unable to pass on any value whatsoever to his family from the practice he had built through many years of hard work.

THE LESSON OF DR. WILLIAMS

Every practice needs a succession plan.

SEEING THE BIG PICTURE

What do each of these tales have in common?

Dedicated, idealistic doctors never grasped the personal fiscal challenges that came with their chosen profession. Nor did they step back to see the full life cycle of their career.

Even worse, no one ever helped these good people understand the basic pillars of personal finance. And, certainly, no one showed them how to strengthen those pillars over time.

In the next chapter, we will look at the six pillars of physician personal finance in some detail. Then, we will learn how to build a structure that can withstand misguided emotions, misinformed friends, self-interested salespeople, and the shifting winds of health-care politics.

CHAPTER FOUR

The Pillars of Wealth Management

You need more than medicine bottles to stay healthy, and you need more than brokerage accounts to stay wealthy. I find it helpful to break wealth management into six basic components, or "pillars." These are as follows:

- Wealth Preservation
- Tax Mitigation
- Asset Protection
- Heir Protection
- Practice Succession
- Charitable Planning

Although not all physicians need all six pillars, nearly every physician needs the first four.

Perhaps you consider yourself financially savvy. I doubt, however, that you can call yourself an expert in all six of my pillars. Indeed, it's likely that you should be using professional services to help you with *all* six—if only because you do not have the time to manage them correctly.

PILLAR I: WEALTH PRESERVATION

Wealth preservation does not mean storing money away in a safe. True wealth preservation can only be accomplished through prudent, evidence-based investment. If all your money stays in cash, inflation alone will cause it to lose 2 to 3 percent in value each year. Indeed, as you age, your investments must grow to create enough ongoing income for you to retire. And believe me, someday you will want to retire.

The next chapter goes into great detail about the science of investing. For now, let me just make a few crucial points.

YOU MUST RECOGNIZE CONFLICTS OF INTEREST

As an investor, you must begin with the understanding that most of the financial industry is built on deeply entrenched conflicts of interest.

Many "financial advisors" are in fact licensed brokers who

are under no legal obligation to put their clients' interests ahead of their own. Their real job is to make as much money as possible from you, as quickly as possible.

This does not mean you can do without financial advice. But as we saw in the cautionary tales, it does mean you must approach all advisors and all their recommendations, with some skepticism. You must develop your own wisdom to evaluate theirs.

YOU MUST REALIZE THAT GOOD INVESTING IS COUNTERINTUITIVE

Second, every good investor must recognize that all investing is deeply counterintuitive.

For example, in most of life, it's safer to follow the crowd, and our brains are wired to instinctively seek safety in the herd. When it comes to investments, however, following the herd often proves dangerous.

We are also wired to think, *Whatever happened this year will probably happen again next year*. This psychological phenomenon is known as the recency effect. As our brain evaluates the possibility of outcomes, we automatically assign more weight to our more recent experiences and less weight to distant memories.

If a crash happened eight years ago, it has already become a distant memory. Therefore, we think it less likely to happen next year. But actually, as time goes on, the chance of a new crash increases.

The recency effect has been studied in detail by Daniel Kahneman, a Nobel Prize-winning psychologist, along with other ways in which our psychology affects our economic decision-making. He asks, in essence, *How is it that people make the same mistakes over and over again?*

Kahneman's recency effect works for both good and bad news. If the most recent event is a stock market rally, then we believe that another rally is imminent—without any evidence to back up our assumption, other than recency.

Another researcher, Terry Odean of the University of California in Berkeley, looked at the way in which the Internet has impacted our investment decision process. He isolated a group of people who did very well in the markets *before* the Internet but obtained little or only mediocre success *after* the arrival of online trading.

Why did that happen? Well, before the Internet, these folks had to call a broker before making a trade.

It wasn't that their brokers were giving them good advice—as we shall see in Chapter 5, most advice from brokers is bad advice. But engaging with their brokers was expensive, perhaps $200 to place a single trade. When each trade cost $200, these investors would think twice, maybe thrice, before making a call. Before the Internet, they traded less frequently, and they traded more prudently.

It's not easy to fight your natural responses, but you must learn to do so. Or, you must work with a financial advisor who will serve as a *brake* on your natural responses.

YOU MUST UNDERSTAND RISK

Any good investor must accept the counterintuitive fact that true prudence requires some risk. Indeed, the often-promoted phrase "riskless investment" represents a contradiction in terms, because *all* investment involves risk. Even a federally insured certificate of deposit brings a deep risk of missed opportunity.

As previously noted, if your money is all in cash, you will automatically give up 2 to 3 percent of your assets' value to inflation each year. In ten years or so, you will have given up 20 to 30 percent of your assets' value. *That makes cash one of the riskiest investments out there*, because it has no upside. However, it does have a guaranteed downside.

Other too-risky behaviors include picking individual stocks and attempting to time the market.

For example, investors often sell a stock and immediately use the money to buy another, "better" stock. Terry Odean collected a massive amount of data on these sell-buy pairs, and he found that on aggregate, *the stock that investors sold outperformed the new stock the investors bought*—by an average of 2 percent a year.

He also found that on aggregate, the more often investors bought and sold, the more money they lost. Hence, the people who paid most attention to the market from day to day did more poorly than those who made long-term investments and let them ride.

In all, research shows that the typical investor gives up about 4 percent a year through poor but easily avoided choices. That means, for example, that an investor could have earned 7 percent over the year through a solid, diversified portfolio held long term. But instead, they earned only 3 percent. With just a small change in investment behavior, they could have substantially changed their lives.

In Chapter 5, I will explain how risk must be measured and controlled in order to preserve your wealth.

YOU MUST RECOGNIZE VOODOO WHEN YOU SEE IT

Perhaps most importantly, you must learn that 90 percent of the investment advice you hear from brokers, Wall Street celebrities, and the media doesn't just include a conflict of interest—it represents *sheer nonsense.*

Call it a malignant kind of voodoo.

You can think about the current state of investing as similar to the state of medicine two hundred years ago. Until the twentieth century, medicine was not a science. It was more of a mystical practice. When people got sick, they went to their priest, shaman, or voodoo practitioner to pray for them or perform a kind of magic. The "doctors" of the time knew nothing about cause and effect, controlled studies, or peer-reviewed papers.

In medieval Europe, these "doctors" would often treat fevers by cutting open a vein and letting out blood. On what basis did they do this? They'd "seen it work" through selective observation. And they could offer their patients high drama. No doubt such techniques killed more people than the fevers themselves.

In the last hundred years, medicine has progressed exponentially—but only by evolving from voodoo to science and from faith to evidence.

Investing is just beginning to develop the kind of rigor and science that medicine developed over the last century. The battle fought by doctors to escape nonsense, hearsay, and chicanery is only now being fought in my own field.

Most of the investment activity found in the brokerages clustered around Wall Street in modern New York City still falls into the realm of voodoo. It's based not on science but on faith. And it's subject to the worst kind of malpractice.

To see voodoo in action, you need look no further than current investment media stars like the famous Jim Cramer. Such people give enormous quantities of advice on their shows with none of it based on serious research. Like the shamans of old, people like Cramer go by their gut feelings—presented with all the drama, faith, and compelling theater of ancient voodoo.

Time after time, these folks' advice has been shown to underperform the general market.

The same can be said of countless brokers, fund managers, technical "charters," trend watchers, and celebrity hedge fund rock stars. They either scoff at investment science or make up a false "science" based on silliness, like chart "double shoulders," "floors," "triple dips," and Fibonacci numbers. Their recommendations are as meaningful as white noise—devoid of useful information.

All these people make a living by promoting the very worst investment techniques: the picking of individual stocks and attempts to time the market.

INVESTMENT SCIENCE DOES EXIST

Starting in the 1960s, however, the advent of the super-computer allowed the academic world to begin creating a true investment science. Thanks to the abundance of data available in the investment world, any theories and practices can now be readily tested against hard historical facts.

A huge body of rigorous research now exists, but it has not been well disseminated to the public. This should not be surprising. Wall Street, in particular, resists investment science, because it proves how most of their practices have no value. Hard-numbers academic research shows that, like bloodletting, much of what passes for expertise on Wall Street destroys more value than it creates—even while that "expertise" makes plenty of money for the experts.

Much of the new science was pioneered by a man named Eugene Fama, who won the Nobel Prize in 2013. We'll look at the work of Fama and his colleague Kenneth French in Chapter 5. We'll also investigate Fama's nemesis, another brilliant academic named Robert Shiller.

BUILDING THE INVESTMENT PILLAR

As we bring this section to a close, let's just summarize.

In order to preserve your wealth, you must build your investment pillar. To build that pillar, you must accept some risk. As you accept risk, you must exercise your medical bias toward evidence-based decisions.

And you must escape the voodoo of the witch doctors.

PILLAR 2: TAX MITIGATION

Most physicians ignore their personal tax issues until they get close to April 15 each year. But your tax situation will always be crucial to your wealth, and it requires careful planning. You should spend some time familiarizing yourself with the fundamental issues, and then you must work with an expert.

PLAN YOUR LIFELONG MOVE FROM LABOR TO CAPITAL

The first thing you have to learn about tax law is that it favors those *with* money, rather than those who merely *earn* money. Learn this lesson young, and you will prosper.

America is a proud capitalist country, where capital gains from invested money are taxed at a much lower rate than labor. The highest long-term capital gains tax rate is 20 percent, while the highest labor tax rate is around 50 percent when you combine state, federal, and other taxes.

This difference is stunning, and it's all-important to your financial well-being. *One of the key goals of your personal finances must be to move from labor to capital over the span of your life and career.*

As I have learned, far too many doctors live paycheck to paycheck throughout their careers, saving nothing despite their high incomes. They think that by working harder they will become richer. But earning more through your labor means paying higher and higher taxes. *Work* harder, and usually the government gets a bigger chunk.

The only sure way to become rich is to use your labor to build a decent capital base as early as possible. Don't spend all your hard-won and heavily taxed earned income. Save your money, and then let it make money for you, *at reduced tax rates.*

As we learned through the example of Rajesh, every young physician should aim for a minimum target of $1 million in investable assets before they start to indulge their desires.

SOME INVESTMENTS ARE TAX EFFICIENT AND SOME ARE NOT

Once you have money to invest, you must begin to consider the tax efficiency of your investments.

Some investments are tax efficient and some are not. The difference is crucial, and it can determine the overall success of your investment strategy. Unfortunately, most people don't give tax efficiency a thought when they start placing their money or making trades. And usually, brokers are all too happy to let their clients ignore the underlying tax issues of major investments.

Here are two simple ideas I want you to understand about investment tax efficiency:

- Investments held for the *long term are taxed much differently* than investments held for less than a year.
- Tax efficiency can be achieved by *locating* your assets in the right kinds of accounts.

LONG-TERM VERSUS SHORT-TERM GAINS

Tax law specifically penalizes short-term gains with higher rates. Generally, this means assets held for less than twelve months.

Short-term capital gains are taxed as regular income, and

the highest federal income tax rate presently stands at 39.5 percent. Just now, there's also an Obamacare surcharge for "rich" folks of 3.8 percent. To that, you can add state income taxes, for a total nearing 50 percent.

If you are in this highest, 50 percent bracket, your short-term gains will be taxed at that same 50 percent.

But long-term capital gains are taxed at only 20 percent and only when realized. In other words, if you hold an investment for twenty years, you will be taxed once in twenty years.

Would you rather pay 50 percent on gains every year, or 20 percent on gains once every twenty or thirty years? It's a no-brainer.

At the individual level, when you make stock market trades, you should always hold an asset for at least a year. Generally, the longer, the better.

Because most of your market assets will be in funds, it also matters a great deal whether your fund manager runs a tax-efficient operation. Do your fund managers churn your funds by buying and selling often, or do they hold individual stocks for the long term?

You can measure fund tax efficiency by looking at the *turn-*

over ratio of a fund. If the turnover ratio is 100 percent, that means the fund manager turns over all its holdings each year. If it's 200 percent, that means they turn it over twice a year, with an average holding period of only six months. If the turnover rate is 10 percent, then the average holding period is ten years.

I look for funds with a turnover rate around 5 percent, which means they hold their investments for twenty years on average.

If you make an investment of $100 in which the baseline return is 8 percent, then in twenty years' time, portfolios holding substantially similar allocations of stocks will show very different returns. Invest your $100 in a fund with tax-efficient investment (low turnover of 5 percent), and it will be worth about $373 after twenty years. The same portfolio invested with low tax efficiency (high churn and turnover of 100 percent or more) will be worth only about $219.

LOCATING YOUR ASSETS PROPERLY

Investment gains come in two forms: investment income and capital appreciation. These are taxed very differently.

Investment income is taxed as personal income every year, in the same way as your labor. Capital gains are taxed only when sold.

Because of this difference, you need to be smart about how you place your investments.

Some investments generate a good deal of annual income but offer low appreciation—for example, a real estate investment trust (REIT). Such investments should be placed in a tax-deferred retirement account, where they will be sheltered from income taxes during your high-income years, with taxes paid only when monies are withdrawn during retirement. After you retire, you will likely be in a lower tax bracket and will pay much lower taxes on your profits.

Assets that provide high appreciation should be put in regular accounts, because they will be held long term anyway, and you will not be taxed on them each year. Again, when you pull these out after retirement, you will likely be taxed at the much lower long-term capital gains rate.

TAX BENEFITS TO PRIVATE PRACTICE

Physicians in private practice have the best chance of earning significant money, but they often neglect the significant tax savings that can come from owning one's own business.

It's beyond the scope of this book to detail all the possibilities, and laws are ever-changing.

If you own your own practice, you should work with a CPA who has specific expertise in medical practice to find these savings, which might include amortizations of equipment, the shifting of income to a real estate holding company for your office, deductions for transportation, and so on.

The Defined-Benefit Plan

One of the best but most frequently missed opportunities of a private practice is the personal defined-benefit plan, which can defer taxes and create what amounts to a personal pension.

Most of us are familiar with defined-contribution plans such as a 401(k) set up by an employer. But a 401(k) severely limits the amount of money you can protect from taxation, currently up to $18,000 a year.

In a defined-benefit plan, rather than defining your annual contribution, you define how much money you want to get in your retirement. You could say, for example, you wish to receive $200,000 a year during your retirement.

To fund that revenue stream, you would need to have about $3 million by the time you retire. To build toward that $3 million, an actuarial expert might calculate that you need to contribute $200,000 into your defined-benefit plan this year and every year while you are working.

Importantly, this $200,000 will be tax deductible.

Setting up a defined-benefit plan is not difficult, but you must utilize a third-party administrator (TPA). Your TPA will then create a plan compliant with the Employee Retirement Income Security Act (ERISA), use actuarial formulas to tell you how much you can contribute each year, and handle the annual reporting with the Department of Labor.

Is such an arrangement worth the effort? Definitely. If you are earning $500,000 or more a year, deferring taxes on $200,000 of that can reap enormous benefits long term and ensure that you retire comfortably.

Exotic Tax Avoidance Schemes

Risky and complicated tax strategies are also available to physicians in private practice. I call these "exotics."

For example, you may toy with the idea of a "captive insurance" program in which you set up a separate insurance company owned by yourself to which you will pay premiums. Because the first million dollars in premiums to a new insurance company are not taxed, a physician can theoretically set up a tax arbitrage in which the premiums are written off by the practice and untaxed at the insurance company.

After many legal battles over such schemes, the Internal Revenue Service (IRS) did establish a safe-harbor ruling in which you can set up a captive insurance company as long as half of its premiums come from a third-party, thus proving you are not simply operating a tax dodge.

Complicated? Yes. Worth the risk? Probably not.

Even if such exotics have been ruled legal, they are usually constructed on the edge of a precipice. Something like captive insurance may be just one legal opinion away from becoming illegal or, at the very least, attracting unwanted IRS attention.

The IRS has already said it will consider any captive insurance scheme as a transaction of interest.

Another exotic tax avoidance strategy is known as the 412(i) insurance pension plan, which was for a long time pushed hard by insurance salespeople as a magical way to cut your income taxes and even your estate taxes. In such a plan, a defined-benefit pension is set up using a complex combination of life insurance and annuities.

Again, the IRS has labeled 412(i) insurance pension plans as transactions of interest.

By labeling something a transaction of interest, the IRS

says that although such a scheme is not, by its nature, illegal, they will look closely, because they have seen many fraudulent arrangements.

In my opinion, exotic tax avoidance schemes are simply not worth the risk and the stress. Often, they assume the IRS is too dumb to figure out what you are doing; but believe me, the IRS is not dumb.

Exotics put you at the edge of a cliff, and you may fall over that cliff without even being aware of falling. Certainly, exotics will require high fees from attorneys, accountants, and insurance agents—fees likely to eat up any tax advantage you would gain.

Use Only a CPA with a Medical Specialty

Tax mitigation should never be an afterthought, even for the busiest physician. And tax mitigation must be delegated. Don't try to do it alone.

As previously noted, you must use a CPA who specializes in medical practices or serves a significant number of physicians. Such a CPA will have a far better chance of staying current with the tax laws most relevant to your profession.

You must also remember you have a right to a CPA, just

as you have a right to an attorney. *If you are ever contacted by the IRS or another tax authority, do not talk to them.* The conversation might head into areas that you have no expertise to discuss, and your words might be used against you. You have every right to tell these authorities to speak only with your CPA.

PILLAR 3: ASSET PROTECTION

Asset protection means preserving your hard-earned wealth from being taken away by others, justifiably or otherwise.

Medicine is a high legal-risk profession. If you are a young physician starting a practice, you have a 96 percent chance of getting sued at least once during your career. According to a recent American Medical Association survey, 5 percent of respondent physicians faced a malpractice claim in the previous year.[1]

The same survey found that not all medical specialties suffer equally. In any given twelve-month period, a neurosurgeon has about a 19 percent chance of being hit by a malpractice suit. An Ob-Gyn has an 11 percent chance. A psychiatrist faces only about a 3 percent chance.

---

[1] Carol K. Kane, "Policy Research Perspectives; Medical Liability Claim Frequency: A 2007–08 Snapshot of Physicians," *American Medical Association* (2010): 1–7.

Physicians with a Malpractice Claim Annually (%)

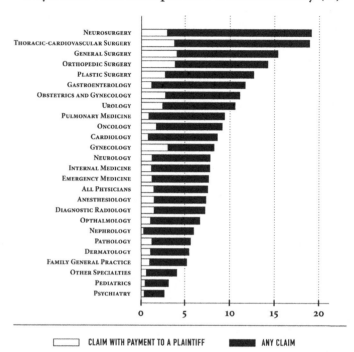

NEUROSURGERY
THORACIC-CARDIOVASCULAR SURGERY
GENERAL SURGERY
ORTHOPEDIC SURGERY
PLASTIC SURGERY
GASTROENTEROLOGY
OBSTETRICS AND GYNECOLOGY
UROLOGY
PULMONARY MEDICINE
ONCOLOGY
CARDIOLOGY
GYNECOLOGY
NEUROLOGY
INTERNAL MEDICINE
EMERGENCY MEDICINE
ALL PHYSICIANS
ANESTHESIOLOGY
DIAGNOSTIC RADIOLOGY
OPTHALMOLOGY
NEPHROLOGY
PATHOLOGY
DERMATOLOGY
FAMILY GENERAL PRACTICE
OTHER SPECIALTIES
PEDIATRICS
PSYCHIATRY

0   5   10   15   20

☐ CLAIM WITH PAYMENT TO A PLAINTIFF   ■ ANY CLAIM

Credit: Medscape[2]

Beyond the disparity of lawsuit odds among different specialties, there's a significant disparity among sexes and ages. Older doctors are more likely to be sued, presumably because they have deeper pockets and make better targets for plaintiff lawyers.

2   Anupam B. Jena et al., "Malpractice Risk According to Physician Specialty," *The New England Journal of Medicine* 365, no. 7 (August 18, 2011), https://www.ncbi.nlm.nih.gov/pmc/articles/PMC3204310/#R14.

One study concluded that while most malpractice suits are without merit, most medical errors do not go to court. The difference appears to come from the "offending" doc's communication skills. A physician with a bad bedside manner may turn a non-mistake into an expensive lawsuit. Male doctors are more likely to be sued, apparently because they are not as good at communicating empathetically with their patients as their female colleagues.

Regardless of the individual statistics or causes, you must accept the fact that you will probably get sued at some point. It's just part of the job.

BUILDING A FORTRESS

Every doctor must, of course, maintain the appropriate level of malpractice insurance. But beyond that insurance, you must also protect your personal assets from attack. You must build a fortress for your money. If opposing attorneys see that you have placed your wealth inside the right kind of fortress, they will often just give up.

If, however, you take no measures beyond insurance to protect your wealth, you will make yourself a more attractive target. If your money is "lying right on the ground," you can be sure that even if you have done nothing to justify lawsuits, you will attract lawsuits.

Let me begin by saying you need professional legal and accounting help to construct your fortress. I can only offer some basic observations.

Foreign Asset Protection Trust

The most secure fortress is a foreign asset protection trust in which you literally move your money outside the country. If you establish a trust in the Bahamas, a US court may render judgment, but the Bahamas will be under no obligation to carry out that judgment.

I do not, however, generally recommend foreign trusts to my clients. Foreign trusts require too much work and are generally not necessary. Unless you have liquid assets totaling over $10 million and face a serious risk, it's unlikely that hiring a specialized, expensive attorney and putting forth considerable effort would be worth it.

Once your assets are moved, you will find it extremely inconvenient to access your money, and it might require continuing legal costs just to maintain that access.

Domestic Asset Protection Trust

The second most secure strategy involves a domestic asset protection trust in which you move your money to a state that provides better protection of assets than your own. Such trusts also involve a good deal of complexity and effort.

You might, for example, consider a trust in Nevada, where current law actually prevents others from learning about your Nevada trust or how much money it contains.

If, however, a plaintiff's attorney does somehow discover your money in Nevada and obtains a judgment against you in another state, Nevada will indeed carry out that other state's court judgment. Some level of secrecy? Yes. Absolute protection such as you can obtain overseas? No.

Once again, you would need to talk to a very good lawyer before attempting to set up a domestic asset protection trust.

Simpler Arrangements

For most physicians, far simpler arrangements can go a long way.

For example, in about half of US states, your assets can be placed in an account structured as "tenants in the entirety" with a spouse. Usually bank accounts are set up only as "joint tenants with rights of survivorship," but mere joint accounts with or without rights of survivorship offer no asset protection and are vulnerable to suits.

Accounts with tenants in the entirety (or similar language) offer the possibility of making your assets inseparable from your spouse's ownership. How does this protect you? Unless your spouse somehow participated in your actual medical mishap, he or she cannot be named in the lawsuit as a defendant, and your joint assets cannot be pulled from the account for a settlement.

Say you are a doctor, and your husband is a flight attendant. You are involved in a medical accident, and the patients sue all the doctors involved. The plaintiff can try to get beyond your malpractice insurance to go after your bank accounts. But if an account has been structured as tenants in the entirety, *your spouse also owns the account in its entirety*. Hence, unless the spouse is actually named as culpable in the lawsuit—for example, he happened to show up in the operating room on a flight layover and handed you a scalpel—this account cannot be attacked.

Obtaining this protection may be as simple as checking the right box when you set up the account. But the precise naming of such accounts, along with the associated protections, varies by state, so you must do your homework. And get the advice of an in-state attorney or accountant.

Here is the present list of states offering tenants in the entirety.[3]

STATES WITH TENANCY BY THE ENTIRETY OF OWNERSHIP	
ALASKA*	MISSOURI
ARKANSAS	NEW JERSEY
DELAWARE	NEW YORK*
DISCTRICT OF COLUMBIA	NORTH CAROLINA*
FLORIDA	OHIO ‡
HAWAII	OKLAHOMA
ILLINOIS**	OREGON*
INDIANA*	PENNSYLVANIA
KENTUCKY*	RHODE ISLAND*
MARYLAND	TENNESSEE
MASSACHUSETTS	VERMONT
MICHIGAN †	VIRGINIA
MISSISSIPPI	WYOMING

* FOR REAL ESTATE ONLY
** FOR HOMESTEAD PROPERTY ONLY
† JOINT TENANCY OF HUSBAND AND WIFE IS AUTOMATICALLY A TENANCY BY THE ENTIRETY
‡ ONLY IF CREATED BEFORE APRIL 4, 1985

Source: NOLO.com

---

3   Mary Randolph, "Avoiding Probate with Tenancy by the Entirety Ownership," *Nolo*, accessed July 14, 2017, http://www.nolo.com/legal-encyclopedia/free-books/avoid-probate-book/chapter6-4.html.

RETIREMENT ACCOUNTS

The different kinds of retirement accounts may or may not offer protection against attack by a plaintiff's attorney.

In general, employer-sponsored plans, such as 401(k), 403(b), and defined-benefit plans, are covered under ERISA and are fully exempt from creditor claims by federal law.

The protections offered by an IRA depend on your state of residence. While most states do protect IRA accounts from creditors, there are a few states that either don't or provide only partial protection.

Again, you must do your homework, work with a qualified in-state attorney or CPA, and make sure your retirement accounts stay protected.

PROTECTING YOUR HOME

You may be shocked to learn that in many states, your personal home may be a highly vulnerable asset in a lawsuit. In other states, your home may be protected from seizure under homestead laws.

As of this writing, Florida, Iowa, Kansas, Oklahoma, South Dakota, and Texas have laws protecting 100 percent of your home's equity—assuming you follow all the rules. Other states may offer limited homestead protection. Some states, such as New Jersey and Pennsylvania, offer no protection at all.

In any case, the amount of protection and the related rules are varied and ever-changing. For example, in New York, the degree of protection changes county by county.

One simple way to protect your home is to take out a home equity loan. Such a loan immediately makes your home a less attractive target, because it is being used as collateral to a bank. The bank holds a lien, *so a plaintiff's lawyer would not just have to fight you but the bank as well.* Suddenly, you have a very strong partner at your side—a partner with an excellent legal staff.

A smart plaintiff's attorney might quickly find it's not worth their effort to fight both you and the bank. Even if they were to win, they know it's likely that not much cash would be realized by taking your home.

Just establishing a home equity line of credit (HELOC) might be sufficient to help protect your home. You don't even need to take any money out through your HELOC.

Again, consult a qualified in-state attorney.

UMBRELLA INSURANCE

Everyone with significant assets should carry an umbrella insurance policy.

Although it will not protect you from medical suits, umbrella insurance will protect you against a wide variety of other liabilities and lawsuits, including things like excessive damages from car accidents.

Umbrella insurance is generally inexpensive and may cost you just $50 a year for $1 million in coverage.

PILLAR 4: HEIR PROTECTION

As a person with significant assets, you have a special responsibility to make sure your spouse, your children, and your other dependents are well taken care of when you pass away.

As I recounted in the introduction, my wealth management business was founded because my own internist passed away, and I was called on to help his surviving family untangle a mess and make the necessary financial adjustments. Again and again, I have witnessed firsthand how poor planning places an enormous and unnecessary legal and emotional burden on loved ones.

UNDERSTANDING THE BASICS

A full discussion of estate planning goes well beyond the scope of this book. But it is crucial to know that you need much more than a mere last will and testament. You also need a qualified estate attorney to draft your documents.

Let's look at a few of the key elements.

The Trust

The first element is the establishment of a trust. Often, the appropriate vehicle is a "living trust," but trusts can take many forms. For example, you may need an A/B trust, which divides into two when one spouse dies. You may need a testamentary trust. Do not assume you understand trusts. Consult a lawyer on the proper type of trust for your individual situation.

And please, do not try to construct a trust on your own, no matter how easy a do-it-yourself Internet site may sound. These templates are not reliable, and they may prove void in your state when the crucial moment arrives.

Once you create a trust, you must move your assets into that trust during your lifetime. When you are alive, you control the trust. Later, control passes to the trustees (usually heirs) you designate.

Without a trust in place, your loved ones will have to go to probate court to establish their rights to your assets, even if you wrote out a last will and testament. This is a difficult, expensive, and time-consuming process at best. And it is not a private process. In probate, personal properties will become public information.

If you have property in multiple states, creating a trust becomes even more important. Without a trust, your loved ones will not only have to go through probate, but they will have to do so in each state, separately.

The Pour-Over Will

The second component is something known as a pour-over will, which makes sure that whatever assets you did not move into your trust will be "poured" into the trust at the moment you die. For example, if you neglected to make your trust the owner of your car, the pour-over will can remedy your oversight. Your heirs will not have to go to court just to get control of your car.

Advance Health-Care Directive

An advance health-care directive says, "If I am incapacitated, these are the instructions to my family and my physicians." Often, this means giving your loved ones permission to end life support if you fall into a vegetative state and cannot make decisions for yourself.

Without such a document, decisions that need to be made by your loved ones will be far more painful. This document also generally gives someone your "durable power of attorney for health-care decisions."

Durable Power of Attorney

You will also need to create a more general durable power of attorney. Despite its confusing title, this document has nothing to do with your attorney. Instead, it gives certain powers to someone you determine, who can conduct business on your behalf if you are incapacitated or even unreachable while out of the country.

Creating a durable power of attorney is certainly crucial if you own your own practice. But everyone should give power of attorney to someone who could, for example, write checks to utilities on their behalf if they were unable to do so themselves.

ELIMINATE UNCERTAINTY

Beyond saving your heirs from the huge hassle of probate, your goal in estate planning must be to *eliminate uncertainty* for your heirs.

Uncertainty creates more than confusion. It consumes energy. And it causes discord.

You will also be protecting the privacy of your heirs, as probate is a public process. Done properly, you can also take substantial steps to save your heirs significant taxes related to your legacy.

MINOR CHILDREN

Anyone with minor children certainly needs estate planning right away. Your will must nominate guardians for young children if something should happen to you and your spouse. Without such a nomination, a court will step in and make its own judgment, possibly placing your children in the care of someone you would not have chosen at all.

You must also deal with the complex questions of how your assets would be handled if you and your spouse were gone but all your children had not reached the age of eighteen.

Often, this means nominating a guardian for the children and a separate guardian for your assets, supervised by the court. Making the proper arrangements in advance will be crucial to ensure honesty and prudence by everyone involved.

Any nominated guardian would have to be approved by a

court at the time of your death, but courts will generally honor a reasonable nomination.

TRANSITIONAL SERVICES AT THE TIME OF CRISIS

You should also consider working with a professional who can provide crucial transitional services to your family in a crisis. An attorney can only advise on legal issues, but good financial advice (and action) at the right moment might mean everything to your loved ones.

People who have suffered a major loss are in no state to process the mountain of paperwork a death or significant incapacity produces—especially the death or incapacity of someone with major assets and responsibilities.

Unfortunately, only the rare financial advisor provides the complete range of services your family might need in such a moment. But when you are interviewing potential advisors, look for someone capable of assuming this burden after you die.

He or she must be proven in this capacity and must care enough about their work to carry the burden properly. You must not, of course, choose someone of your own age or older, who may themselves be retired or have passed on when they are needed most.

WHEN DO YOU ACTUALLY NEED LIFE INSURANCE?

Often, I find that physicians have completely neglected estate planning but have purchased hefty life insurance policies, thinking they have now protected their heirs.

Like most people, these doctors usually have a confused understanding of life insurance. Not surprisingly, this confusion is fostered by the lucrative insurance industry.

Often, people see life insurance as an investment product or a form of asset protection.

Insurance *can* play a vital role in protecting your heirs when young. It can also play a vital role in practice partnerships.

But as we saw in the cautionary tales of Dr. Edwards and Dr. Chang, physicians are often targeted by insurance agents for the wrong type of insurance. Often, these permanent policies are very, very expensive and cover the wrong kinds of risks—even nonexistent risks—while creating lifelong monetary obligations.

Let me make this as clear as possible: *Life insurance is a contract to hedge against the financial risk to dependent heirs in the event of the untimely death of their financial provider*—with emphasis on the word *untimely*. In the context of one's family, it should serve no other purpose.

As of this writing, I have two young children, eight and five. When they were born, I bought a $500,000 term life insurance policy on myself, to benefit my wife and kids if I died suddenly. Because I was young and healthy, it cost me just $150 a quarter, about $600 a year. I did not see this insurance as an investment; I saw it as managing risk.

If I educate my children well, when they reach maturity, they will not be dependent on me financially anymore. Hence, I will no longer need life insurance to protect them. Put simply, term life insurance for the first twenty to twenty-five years of a child's life is important—*a limited term during which I must pay premiums.* After that, it can play no useful role.

Of course, if a child has special needs, he or she may always be a dependent, in which case, I do help my clients shop for whole life insurance (see the sections that follow)—one of the rare occasions in which permanent policies make sense.

Insure a Child's Life? Seriously?

Incredibly, as we learned in the case of Dr. Chang, sometimes an insurance agent will sell a policy on a *child's life.* This is absurd, as your children have no dependents.

Working adults who support themselves are sometimes

even talked into insuring their parents' lives, at high cost—a very poor investment and a hedge against a nonexistent risk.

To protect a nonworking spouse, you should carry *term life insurance* until you accumulate enough assets so your spouse could survive comfortably if you had an untimely death. Indeed, at the risk of sounding cavalier, a young, educated spouse with job skills or the capacity to remarry would likely find another way to survive without a hefty insurance payout.

Whole Life, Universal Life, and Permanent Life Policy Scams

Permanent life is a broad term that includes both whole life and universal life insurance policies. Either way, this insurance is designed to persist through your entire life. For most people, that means long after it's needed.

Whole life contracts are rigorous. You must pay certain premiums your entire life, with a specific, promised death benefit when you die. Fail to make the payments each month, *and you risk losing your entire investment.* In what other investment vehicle must you play such a danger-ous game?

Universal life offers more flexibility, but it often proves an even worse deal. With universal life, you can say, "This month, I cannot pay so much, so I'll pay less. A few months from now, I'll catch up." However, the contract also gives the insurance company more flexibility, potentially allowing them to play games with your benefits and wriggle out of the deal. You should not be surprised that insurance companies have structured these contracts so the advantage usually flows to them.

An Especially Bad Universal Life Deal

For example, I had a client whose father had bought a universal life insurance policy twenty-three years earlier. The premium was $10,000 a year, with a promised death benefit of just $500,000. Over those twenty-three years, the father had paid out a total of $230,000. But despite that the insurance company had been using and investing that money for more than two decades, the "cash value" of the policy was only $150,000. Meaning, if he withdrew the money immediately, that's all the father would receive.

But the story gets much worse. This universal life insurance policy allowed the company to charge a "mortality cost" against the cash value, levied each year. When the father bought the policy, he was just fifty-two. Now he was seventy-five, and because his chance of dying had risen considerably, so did the "mortality cost"—hitting $50,000 a year. Of that money, $10,000 was coming out of the premium, and $40,000 was coming out of the cash value of the policy. What does that mean? In under four years, this $40,000 charge would have completely destroyed the cash value, and when the cash value was gone, the policy would have lapsed. In other words, the approximately $270,000 paid into this so-called "permanent life" policy would have been given to the insurance company as a gift.

Only if the father died in less than four years would the son receive any death benefit at all. Hard to believe, but true.

I managed to renegotiate the policy, reducing the death benefit to $300,000, hence lowering the mortality cost. In that way, the $10,000 annual premium, if paid, would continue to support the policy for another fifteen years. But it remained a staggeringly bad deal.

Insurance agents try to sell young parents whole life or universal life policies on the theory that these are long-term retirement investments and some kind of fund for their children's futures. In truth, however, permanent life policies are usually terrible investments that manage the wrong kind of risk.

Indeed, such policies generally hedge against a risk that does not exist.

Why do agents push these bad deals? Because whenever an

agent lands a new permanent life contract, they typically take home 100 percent of the first year's premium themselves—$10,000, in the case above. After that, the agent usually receives 3 to 5 percent a year for as long as the contract is in force, which might mean the rest of your life. Of course agents push these big packages and lifetime commitments!

As previously noted, for my clients who have children with special needs, I often help them shop for a whole life policy, *as opposed to universal life*. Twenty-five years from now, the child will still be a dependent, and possibly even forty years from now. At least, with whole life, the contract will rigorously ensure that the insurance company fulfills its end of the bargain. The company will be locked in, not just my client.

In most cases, however, the enormous sums of money dropped into a permanent life insurance policy should instead be invested properly for the future of both the doctor and the doctor's family.

Insuring the Life of a Practice Partner

Another important use of whole life insurance involves private-practice partnerships.

If I am in a coequal business partnership with another

doctor, and we both have a spouse, what happens if one of us dies? Without an appropriate buy/sell agreement backed by insurance, the spouse of the deceased partner would become the new coequal partner in the practice, even though he or she had no experience in medicine or in business.

A good business partnership will include a buy/sell agreement with a provision for an insurance settlement to buy out the surviving spouse. Suppose the business has a total value of $2 million. If one of the business partners dies, the surviving partner would get $1 million from a whole life insurance policy, with the mandatory provision that he or she must purchase the other half of the business, and the surviving spouse must sell.

The insurance itself will be a deductible business expense with a tax benefit. If the partnership has a known termination date, then the business would buy term life instead of whole life.

Never Buy More Insurance Than You Need

The bottom line on insurance? Never carry more than you need. You should evaluate your risk on a regular basis, and you should seek advice from an independent financial advisor, not an insurance agent with an inherent conflict of interest.

PILLAR 5: PRACTICE SUCCESSION

Most private physicians work *in* their practices; they don't work *on* their practices.

Few physicians in private practice do the right kind of planning for the day they retire. Such planning must begin far in advance. Most experts advise at least five years of forward thinking and preparation, even ten.

With the right succession planning, you can capture the equity value in a private practice, and you can ensure a smooth transition for your patients on the day you retire. Indeed, the right planning can improve your practice and your livelihood long before you retire.

Without proper succession planning, your patients will scatter when you retire or become incapacitated. When that occurs, your practice's inherent value—the equity and goodwill represented by your practice—will be lost. Indeed, once patients see you are nearing retirement, they may begin looking for other doctors, rapidly diminishing the value of your life's work. Far too often, doctors realize nothing or next to nothing on practices they have built up over decades.

By failing to plan, you are also not taking good care of your patients. They will lose continuity of care and be left to their own devices in finding a new physician. Far too many doctors simply coast to the end, letting their roster of patients diminish and ceasing to enroll new patients, until one day they just take down their shingle.

Coasting now carries a new kind of risk. Changing health-care laws require that medical records be retained for five to ten years. So, retired doctors may find themselves acting as full-time record keepers, pulling out old files for old patients, well after the shingle comes down. If no one has purchased your practice, the responsibility will fall on you. As health-care laws shift, those responsibilities and their related liabilities are likely to increase, not decrease, over time.

THE CHALLENGES

I should begin by saying that physician private practices usually sell for lower multiples than other small businesses. As of this writing, medical practices typically realize only in the range of 0.3 to 0.7 times annual revenues. Dental offices do much better, at 1 to 1.5 times revenues. Other kinds of small business, including a financial advisory like mine, often realize 2 to 4 times gross annual revenue.

Why the low values for private practices? Because health care is a highly regulated industry with a good deal of uncertainty.

Patients may not stick with a new doctor or medical group. The practice may carry forward liability. And the political party in Washington may change within a year or two, bringing with it a whole new idea of how to fund health care, which could upset the economic basis of the practice.

Investors figure all this uncertainty into the price.

FOUR BASIC ROADS TO SUCCESSION

That said, there are many ways to increase the value of your practice and ensure that you get the best possible price.

I see four basic roads to selling a private medical practice. Each has its advantages and disadvantages. Not all will be possible for certain specialties and situations. High-demand specialties such as ophthalmology, dermatology, and emergency medicine will offer the most options. Family practices, pediatric practices, and Ob-Gyn are less well received in the market. The larger your office in terms of number of physicians, the more attractive, and valuable, it will become.

You should choose and actively pursue one of the roads listed here, allowing for fallback options. And you should review your plan with experts, updating it as the marketplace and politics of health care demand.

Below, I rank the possibilities in terms of expected profitability.

- Sell your practice to a private equity firm currently consolidating services in your specialty or geography.
- Hire an associate doctor and groom him or her for succession. At some point, the associate doctor(s) can take over, gradually paying you off for your personal equity in the organization.
- Sell your practice to another doctor in independent practice.
- Sell your practice to an existing, larger medical organization, such as a hospital or group.

Each of these methods will allow you to capture some of the value you created, while also providing good continuity of care for your patients. Let's discuss each briefly.

Private Equity

Private equity firms offer the most lucrative possibilities for a sale, because they are actively pursuing strategies in specific specialties and looking to merge practices to realize cost savings and boost profits. They also want to cut deals with insurance companies and move into specific disease management opportunities.

These firms are often only interested in specific specialties, but if you are a fit, you can tailor your practice to their needs and potentially get top dollar.

Grooming a Successor

Your second most lucrative option will be to hire one or two associate doctors with the intention of grooming them for future succession. This requires working out a long-term deal in which the other doctors buy up your equity over time, eventually taking control of the entire practice.

Even if the succession is never completed, a larger practice will become much more attractive to private equity groups and others, offering a more stable patient base and lower risk.

Of course, the grooming process rarely proves simple. For starters, you have to find a younger doctor who shares your medical philosophy and who fits with both your personality and the expectations of your patients. A doctor with aggressive treatment philosophies will not fit with a doctor who prefers to suggest changes to diet and exercise habits. The new doc must also be carefully introduced to the existing patient roster and must learn to bring in new patients of his or her own to make it all pencil out.

Typically, the new doctor will be hired simply as an

employee for a year or two to see if there's a fit before an offer is made for a long-term partnership and buyout. At that point, lawyers and practice advisors must be brought in, as the terms will be complex.

Grooming a successor is a complicated road with plenty of pitfalls. Indeed, doctors often find the whole thing too daunting and never start looking for an associate, or they give up after a couple of tries.

But persistence pays off.

For years, I pestered one of my clients, let's call him Dr. Mussaf, to hire an associate and begin the succession process. When he finally started, it took him two years to locate the right associate, and the first year created a lot of stress within the practice. But in the second year, Dr. Mussaf told me the arrangement had really begun to pay off. His profit increased 30 percent, and the time he worked went down 20 percent. Within three years, the new doc was generating just as much volume as Dr. Mussaf, but the overhead in staff, equipment, and space had increased only 10 percent.

Indeed, when I meet with Dr. Mussaf, I now find him looking much healthier. He has time to exercise and play tennis. And he tells me he is a happier man.

Importantly, once you have hired the first associate, you will find it much easier to hire the second and the third. You will understand the process, you will have put the mechanisms in place, and the culture of your office will have adjusted to the idea of multiple physicians.

Selling to Another Independent Physician

Simply selling your practice to another independent doctor in your own specialty rarely produces a good price, and it may be fraught with difficulties.

The buyer will be rightly concerned that patients will not accept a new doctor they have never met and will simply disappear when you retire. Your medical records system may be incompatible, your paper records may be indecipherable, and both may be loaded with potential liability that an independent doctor cannot handle.

As a result, even if you find an independent buyer of this kind, he or she will generally look for a huge discount on your equity.

Selling to a Hospital or Other Large Group

Probably the least profitable way of exiting from your practice will be to sell out to a hospital and become a short- or long-term employee. Large groups present similar issues.

This may, of course, be your only option if you have not groomed a successor; and selling to a big medical organization may offer the least hassle and liability, even if you realize little of your equity in the process.

There was a time, of course, when hospitals rarely hired physicians. Hospitals served only as the meeting ground for patient and doctor, providing the underlying infrastructure of beds, nurses, and equipment. But as hospitals move toward becoming complete health-care providers, even managed-care providers, they have begun hiring lots of docs.

This process has been greatly accelerated by changes in the health-care system such as the ACA, which introduced enormous burdens of record keeping and administration. This made it more and more difficult for doctors to function independently.

These laws also provided huge incentives for hospitals to become part of what are known as Accountable Care Organizations (ACOs). It's a complex subject, but basically, hospitals join with other providers to participate in a Medicare fee-for-service incentive program. ACOs are paid to reduce costs by creating overall healthy outcomes for their patients. The net result? Less value in independent practices.

This trend is likely to continue.

When a hospital acquires your practice, it will see you merely as a new employee. You may get a salary boost in the first one or two years to compensate you for the equity they acquired, but this bonus will not be anything close to the value you might have realized by following one of the other roads I described. In a large medical group, you may or may not have the opportunity to become a partner and participate in greater equity over time.

At a certain point, of course, the pressures of your own practice may have become too great. You may not have another viable plan, and you may be ready to become just an employee.

OTHER CONSIDERATIONS

Preparing any practice for sale requires thinking through numerous opportunities and pitfalls—a subject much too large for this book.

For example, if your practice has not fully converted from paper records to EMR, it will be worth considerably less and may even be unsellable. If patient information is not readily available and cannot be easily integrated into larger data systems, that information may be useless to others and will create too much liability for *any* buyer.

Other considerations may include the real estate that

houses your practice. If you own the building, it may be in your best interest to retain ownership after the sale and derive long-term income from leasing the space to your former practice.

And of course, you will add considerable value to any sale if you agree to stay on for a transitional period of one or two years and introduce your patients to new doctors. You may also be valuable as a marketing tool to a new group or even a hospital.

All these issues require serious legal and business advice. Start early in finding the right help and consult with practice succession experts regularly as you pursue all available options.

PILLAR 6: CHARITABLE PLANNING

Not every physician develops a serious charitable inclination. I find that about a third of the physicians I work with tell me they want to make a significant charitable impact during their lives.

Many of these have accumulated more than $5 million in assets. But lots of physicians, when they grow older and more financially secure, become more charitable. They begin to see the larger meaning of their lives, and that meaning often lies outside of their personal interest.

Unfortunately, few of these doctors understand how *long-term* charitable planning can dramatically save on taxes during their high-income years while maximizing their charitable impact later on.

For most people, their high-income years do not coincide with their giving years. Your forties and fifties are usually your high-income years. But people generally become more charitable once they retire, have time for charitable work, and know that they're financially secure. That's why the charitable years usually come during a doctor's sixties and seventies.

As we learned with Dr. Farooq, if you see your life moving in this arc, it's important to take action to maximize your impact and realize the tax benefits early on.

THE DONOR-ADVISED FUND

If charitable foundations are for the super wealthy, folks like Bill Gates and Warren Buffet, a donor-advised fund is for the merely wealthy and not so wealthy. It's convenient, easy to set up, and easy to administer.

I typically use a donor-advised fund to help my physician clients save taxes now as well as save for their future charitable donations. With this vehicle, your actual donations may not occur until twenty years from now, but the tax benefits can be realized today, when you're in your highest tax bracket.

A donor-advised fund works like a simple version of a charitable foundation. Once it's created, you can, for example, donate $10,000 to the fund every year. The $10,000 is deductible in that same year, even though it has only gone into the fund and not yet to a specific nonprofit. You may choose to give away $3,000 of that money this year, but the other $7,000 will stay in the fund and grow until you are ready to give it to a charity, perhaps during your retirement.

If you set up no fund, and you wait to make these donations when you are in your sixties and seventies, *you will have no significant income against which to take a deduction.* That means you've lost some of the most important write-offs you might ever have taken.

Any large, reputable investment company like Fidelity or Vanguard can set up a donor-advised fund for you. In addition, a financial advisor can find other ways for you to maximize both deductions and contributions.

For example, when I contribute to my own donor-advised fund, I usually contribute an appreciated asset like a stock. In that way, I can avoid capital gains taxes, but I still get the full amount of the tax deduction for the full value of the stock. Both the charity and I become winners.

Suppose I bought a stock for $5,000, and it increased 100 percent over time, so it's now worth $10,000. If I sell the stock and then contribute the money, I will have to pay about 20 percent or $1,000 in capital gains tax. Then I can donate only $9,000 to the charity.

If, on the other hand, instead of selling the stock, I donate it to my donor-advised fund, I avoid the $1,000 in capital gains taxes, and I have provided $10,000 in value to the fund. In addition, because my combined federal and state tax rate is almost 50 percent, I will get about $5,000 in tax deductions. Net result? I gave away $10,000 in charity and saved about $6,000 in taxes.

With my donor-advised fund, I almost feel as if I have my own charitable foundation—and it's a great feeling.

Even if you don't see yourself planning for big donations later in life, you may be giving pretty regularly to a church, a synagogue, a mosque, or another nonprofit. Sitting down with a good financial advisor and tax planner can properly leverage these donations and maximize their effect.

FOCUSING OUR ATTENTION

In this chapter, we saw how every physician must look at the big picture and get the right advice on all aspects of his or her personal finances.

But we also learned the most important pillar is a solid investment strategy. Without such a strategy, the other pillars become irrelevant, wealth preservation becomes impossible, and the most carefully built financial house will collapse.

That's why the next chapter will drill down on investment science.

CHAPTER FIVE

Investment Science

As a physician who believes in evidence-based science, peer-reviewed approaches to treatment, and controlled clinical studies, you may find the title of this chapter hard to accept.

Your financial investments really can be approached with scientific rigor. You really can move past the voodoo practiced by Wall Street and the false investment media "gurus."

My personal story in investment science began in 1992, when I was a graduate student in financial economics at Carnegie Mellon. I was studying for a PhD. It was an exciting time, as in June of that same year Eugene Fama, aided by his colleague Kenneth French, published "The Cross-Section of Expected Stock Returns," one of the most influential papers ever written in finance.

Twenty-one years later, Fama would share the 2013 Nobel Prize in Economics, and the implications of his work would continue to spread, despite the threat his work represented to the witch doctors of the investment world.

Like many of my fellow students, I read Fama as a revelation. At the time, I had no idea that I would someday become a financial advisor implementing the ideas of his seminal paper. But I knew I was seeing a true science of investing finally being created—right before my eyes.

THREE BIG IDEAS YOU SHOULD UNDERSTAND

In this chapter, I want to lay out three simple concepts underlying investment science that have influenced my financial career and should influence all your personal investment decisions.

As a scientist yourself, I think you'll appreciate a little background and evidence for these big ideas. Along the way, I'll summarize the "made easy" investment best practices that result from the science.

The first two concepts are grounded in the work of Fama, and the third comes from Fama's rival, Robert Shiller, who also won a Nobel Prize for Economics in that same year of 2013. Once you understand the thinking of these men, you will feel far more comfortable in the stock market, and you will never fall prey to voodoo investing again.

The three concepts are as follows:

- The Efficient Market Hypothesis: There's No System to Beat the System
- The Smart Banker: How Risk Relates to the Size and Value of Companies
- "Animal Spirits:" How to Recover from a Major Market Crash

CONCEPT 1: THE EFFICIENT MARKET HYPOTHESIS

Fama's famous hypothesis grew from his own work as a PhD student back in 1960. His professor had asked him to find a trading rule that would guarantee an investor would make money. In other words, "Find a system to beat the system." Fama was a student with an assignment from his professor, so he got to work.

The future Nobel winner began by testing many of the trading rules people had put forth in the past. Once he checked these against the actual data of market results, however, he found that the rules put forth in one year almost always failed in the next year. Wait long enough, and all the rules failed.

Why was that?

Fama asked himself, *What if no rule can possibly exist that will consistently beat the market? What if such a rule is theoretically impossible?*

And then he had his insight.

All the proposed trading rules were based on analyzing existing data to predict the future, *but whatever information the trading rule used, the market already knew as well.* Hence, that information could not actually be used to outperform the market, because the market would already have taken it into account.

THE ARAB PRINCE IN GRAND CENTRAL STATION

Let's make the Efficient Market Hypothesis a bit less abstract.

Suppose an Arab prince shows up in New York's Grand Central Station one day at noon with a bag full of $100 bills. He empties the bag from an upper staircase, and immediately, hundreds of people go running around, grabbing the money. It's gone in less than thirty seconds. No one knew he was coming, and only a lucky few get any cash.

No one knows about the event in advance, and the people who learn about the event even thirty seconds late get nothing at all.

The next day at precisely noon, the same thing happens. The same Arab prince shows up and empties a bag of bills. Once again, there's a riot. Once again, a lucky few get the money. Once again, most people are seconds too late.

Naturally, come the third day, precisely at noon, twenty-five thousand people are standing under the staircase waiting. They think they have found the secret rule of the marketplace—the pattern guaranteed to make them money.

And indeed, even on the third day, the Arab prince shows up! He tosses the money! But now the crowd is so great that, again, only a lucky few manage to grab any money. *The market has efficiently absorbed the data and reset the odds just as they were.*

On the fourth day, a hundred thousand people show up at noon. But, oops! The Arab prince decides not to show up until 4:00 p.m., and so it goes.

At the most basic level, the hypothesis says you cannot use a past stock price to predict a future stock price.

So clear has this truth become that you now read this

statement on just about every piece of marketing material you get from an investment house and on just about every monthly statement they mail to you.

If the market becomes briefly inefficient, such as when some basic trading rule changes, it quickly reestablishes its efficient use of information. And if you *were* able to miraculously discover a rule that made you money for a few months—such as by being there at 2:00 a.m. for an Arab prince—others would quickly discover that rule and get there before you.

BUT THE VOODOO GOES ON

Even though Fama proved that market timing of individual stocks, even the overall market, is impossible, you will still find many people whose livelihood depends on making up bogus *timing rules*. These folks look at a chart of a stock or a market index's past performance and then tell you where it's headed next.

These charters will show you resistance levels, breakthrough levels, double shoulders, triple shoulders, and the like. They will tell you with great confidence that if a price hits a resistance level three times and does not break through, then the price is going to drop big. Or rise. Et cetera.

With computer analysis of long-term data, it's easy to demonstrate that shoulders, resistance level, and all the rest are utterly meaningless. The Efficient Market Hypothesis says that what the charters tell you is basically random information—*useless*. When they show you data proving their formula, they are *always* drawing the target after firing the arrow.

The same is true of the gut voodoo practiced by media superstars. I personally examined Jim Cramer's top picks in 2008. By year's end, *all* of them had underperformed the broad S&P 500 Index regardless of the entertainment value of his high-pitched voice.

PRIVATE INFORMATION IS DIFFERENT

But what about private information? What about secret, insider knowledge about specific companies or upcoming legal decisions? Over the years, researchers have proven that, yes, people with private information, such as US senators or officers of public companies, can indeed beat the market.

When CEOs buy and sell their own stock, they tend to do it at a very good time—in essence, timing the market in a way no one else can. They know precisely when the Arab prince will next arrive.

CONCEPT 2: THE SMART BANKER REWARDS RISK

The Efficient Market Hypothesis does not rule out wise investing by people without insider knowledge. On the contrary, it can help ensure wise investing. How? By clear-headed data analysis.

Back when he published his original paper, Fama took all the stock market data from 1963 to 1990, including every public stock. It was a huge amount of data, but by 1992, the computing power was available to deal with it. Rather than looking at individual stocks, he asked, *How do stock prices behave in aggregate?*

In other words, if we ignore voodoo, what can we really see happening?

SMALL IS BETTER THAN LARGE? YOU MUST BE KIDDING

Fama found something very interesting. He found that on average, and completely contrary to what everyone believed, *small-cap stocks outperformed large-cap stocks in the long run.*

In academic terms, we say small-cap stocks have higher *expected returns* than large-cap stocks. Following is the original chart from the seminal paper by Fama and French, covering the period from 1963 to 1990.[4]

Annual Returns Relative to Size

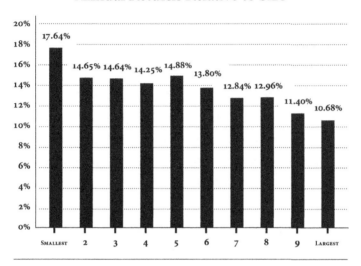

The chart covers all stocks in the market every year from 1963 to 1990, divided into ten deciles according to market capitalization. On the y-axis, we see the average return of each decile over those twenty-eight years. *Yup, small companies did better.*

4   Eugene F. Fama and Kenneth R. French, "The Cross-Section of Expected Stock Returns," *The Journal of Finance* 47, no. 2 (June 1992), http://faculty.som.yale.edu/zhiwuchen/Investments/Fama-92.pdf.

GROWING COMPANIES DO WORSE THAN NONGROWING?

Fama and French also found that—again, totally contrary to popular belief—*nongrowing companies had better returns than growing companies.* Put in academic terms, they found that "value companies" have higher expected returns than "growth companies."

When we talk about a growth company, we mean something like Facebook. It has very little book value. It owns perhaps only a few buildings, desks, and some computer equipment. Indeed, Facebook may even rent most of their buildings and not own them.

A good example of a value company would be a railroad. Its book value includes its freight cars, passenger cars, engine cars, rail yards, warehouses, and so on. All these assets may be very expensive, but the company's stock price will probably not be that high. A railroad company probably experiences little or no growth, so people price it very cheaply.

Even though most of us tend to focus on the Facebooks and Googles of the world, the *vast majority of growth companies actually do not deliver a high return.* If you group the growth companies together and average out their returns, you actually find that value companies do better over time.

Indeed, you will find that the famous investor Warren Buffet tends to invest in railroad companies, furniture stores, paint stores, and other "boring" stocks. He tends to invest in value companies, and he has become one of the richest people on earth.

Here's the original chart from Fama and French[5], again covering returns from 1963 to 1990. The price-to-book (P/B) ratio has been used as a valuation measure. High P/B stocks are called the "growthest" stocks, and low P/B stocks are "valuest" stocks. Again, all market stocks are divided into deciles.

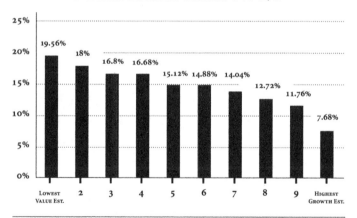

5   Fama and French, *Journal of Finance* 47, no. 2.

To this day, most people prefer bigger companies over smaller ones, and most people believe a high-growth company is sure to deliver high returns.

Why aren't they right? Fama says it's all about *risk*. His argument is a little difficult to grasp at first, so bear with me.

Fama argued that the stock market *generally* rewards the taking of risk. He then goes on to argue that the risk in buying small company stocks is higher than the risk in buying large company stocks—and that risk is rewarded.

In the same way, the risk in buying the stock of a nongrowing value company is higher than the risk in buying the stock of a growth company. Hence, on average, the small companies and value companies provide greater returns over time.

I said that good investment science requires a lot of counterintuitive thinking! When you try to convince people of these statements, they usually look at you like you've lost your mind.

Another Nobel winner, Merton Miller, explained these same ideas in a way that might make them clearer.

Miller once told an audience to imagine the stock market

as a very smart banker. Now suppose you are that smart banker, and two companies come to you to borrow $1 million. Suppose one is Facebook, and the other is the furniture store down the road. Facebook is growing very fast, and the furniture store is growing very slowly or not growing at all—maybe even shrinking.

When these two companies come to borrow $1 million from you, *which one will you charge the higher interest rate to?*

Most people would answer by saying they would charge the furniture store a higher interest rate. Why? Because lending money to a fast-growing company is not risky, but lending money to a slow-growing, nongrowing, or shrinking company is risky indeed. Before lending this furniture store any money, I would demand a very high interest rate—maybe triple of what I'd charge Facebook.

Miller says that the market is acting like a smart banker—essentially demanding a higher return on investment, a "higher interest rate," from slow-growing companies. And the market gets what it demands.

The same can be said for small companies versus large companies. If you want to get a higher return, you have to take more risk, and the market is astoundingly smart in rewarding that risk. Like value companies, small companies are riskier investments, so they provide more returns, *on average, over time.*

DATA PROVEN AGAIN AND AGAIN

People have done similar research on markets in Europe and Asia, and they have found the same pattern of returns. Indeed, the same research has been repeated for the market returns since 1990 with identical conclusions.

At this point, we can say these charts represent a general character of the market. And by 2013, these theories were sufficiently proven to merit the Nobel Prize.

DOES THIS KNOWLEDGE CONTRADICT THE HYPOTHESIS?

"But wait," the reader may object at this point. "If you can predict the market based on the size of companies and their P/B ratios, aren't you violating the Efficient Market Hypothesis? I mean, if everyone has this knowledge, then it's useless, right?"

The answer is simple. This knowledge does not contradict the hypothesis; indeed, it validates the hypothesis, because it shows that the market is efficiently using all information and *efficiently rewarding risk on average and over time.*

According to Fama, the market is in a relentless drive

toward efficiency. If a market feature lasts only a few days or a few months, you can be sure it's just a temporary inefficiency. If a market feature persists for many decades and in all stock markets, then it's not an inefficiency—it represents risk. That's why the Nobel committee waited two decades to give Fama the Nobel Prize.

So, you can indeed use this information to do some scientific investing.

APPLYING CONCEPTS 1 AND 2 IN MY INVESTING PRACTICE

How do I put these two vital concepts to work in my investment strategies? It's very simple.

- The first rule is to avoid actively trading individual stocks, because it is literally impossible to time trades correctly.
- When possible, have a tilt toward small-cap, value stocks.
- Avoid funds that employ active money managers, and instead put money into passively managed index or asset-class funds. Indeed, in an average year:

Twenty-five percent of all money managers outright lose money picking stocks. Seventy-five percent of all money managers make some money, but not enough to overcome their costs.

Only a miniscule 0.24 percent of money managers beat the market by picking individual stocks. There's absolutely no way to predict who will be these lucky few in any upcoming year.

CONCEPT 3: "ANIMAL SPIRITS" AND SURVIVING A CRASH

"OK," you might say. "After reading all of the above, I believe you. I'll stop trying to pick stocks, and I'll stop reading the daily financial prognosticators. I see why I should invest long term, *but what if the whole market crashes?*"

To fully understand the stock market—and to protect against a major market crash—I must introduce the ideas of that other 2013 Nobel Prize winner, Robert Shiller.

Shiller looked at the vast store of stock market data in a different way than Fama, and he came to a radically different conclusion. He said that rather than just looking at company size and value, we should be focusing on *dividends*. Dividends are the yearly payouts to investors who own stock—sometimes substantial, sometimes zero.

In essence, Shiller made the following argument, which I paraphrase: "When you buy a stock, what you get is the future dividend stream; so logically speaking, as the dividend moves, so should the price."

But when this future Nobel Prize winner graphed dividend prices against stock prices over the years, there *at first appeared to be no relationship at all between the two lines of data.*

The dividends were highly stable, but the prices ran up and down like crazy. In his chart, average dividends, normalized for inflation, are shown on the dotted line. Normalized stock prices are shown on the solid line.[6]

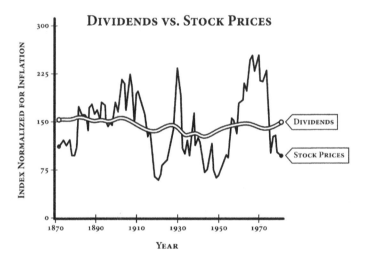

His conclusion? Never mind risk/reward or efficient use of information. Stock prices are driven by *emotion*, or what

---

6   Robert J. Shiller, "Do Stock Prices Move Too Much to be Justified by Subsequent Changes in
    Dividends?" National Bureau of Economic Research, working paper no. 456 (February 1980),
    http://www.nber.org/papers/w0456.pdf.

Shiller called "animal spirits." Nothing else could explain this wild gyration.

Sometimes we get excited, and sometimes we get crazy excited. When we're "exuberant," we drive the price way above the intrinsic value of a stock. When we're pessimistic, even for no apparent reason, we will push the price way below its intrinsic value.

Shiller's famous book *Irrational Exuberance* was published in March 2000, at the very height of the market bubble, which burst shortly thereafter.

Forget that "smart market" stuff from Fama, says Shiller, who famously remarked, and again I paraphrase: "Gene Fama is a good friend of mine who believes in a different religion." In Shiller's view, market forces, like people, are basically irrational, driven by fear and greed. That means prices will always alternate between underpricing and overpricing.

APPLYING SHILLER'S INSIGHTS AFTER A CRASH

The second time you look at Shiller's graph of volatility versus earnings, you will see that regardless of the wild swings of stock prices, you actually *can* find a relationship between the two lines.

Look closely, and you will see that *the market does generally return to its intrinsic value*, as represented by the normalized dividends—*at least over time.*

We can use that knowledge to plan for the worst. For starters, if the market crashes by 80 percent tomorrow, you should not panic. Why? Because the price you pay has crashed, but the value you will receive has not. Although dividends dip, *dividends have never to date "crashed" at all.*

Now, what precisely should you do if the market crashes?

Shiller's insight suggests an answer: *Buy high-dividend stocks at the new, cheaper prices, and reinvest the dividends. Indeed, when the market crashes, it's the perfect time to purchase these stocks.*

DIVIDEND STOCKS TO THE RESCUE

I ran an investment model inspired by Shiller through the Great Depression of the 1930s. As a financial advisor, I asked myself, *What would have been the right way to manage my client's money during the Great Depression, assuming I did not see it coming?*

At one point during the Great Depression, the market actually dropped 87 percent. If I had been there in the

1930s, what should I have done with my clients' money to help them recover?

To do the analysis, I constructed four theoretical portfolios for the Great Depression. Each portfolio had a different mix of dividend-producing stocks, purchased right before the crash.

DIVIDEND TO RESCUE

1. **PORTFOLIO A**: Stocks with zero dividends.
2. **PORTFOLIO B**: Stocks with bottom 30% dividend yields.
3. **PORTFOLIO C**: Stocks with middle 40% dividend yields.
4. **PORTFOLIO D**: Stocks with top 30% dividend yields.

All four portfolios peaked in August, 1929. With the exception of portfolio B, all portfolios bottomed in May, 1933. Portfolio B bottomed in June, 1933. For each of the four portfolios, the total peak-to-trough decline (drawdown) and the number of months it took to recover are presented here:

BUY AT THE TOP AND HOLD DURING GREAT DEPRESSION				
	A	**B**	**C**	**D**
DRAWDOWN	89%	86%	85.4%	84%
MONTHS TO RECOVER	132	154	144	44

DATA SOURCE: KENNETH FRENCH DATA LIBRARY

Only Portfolio D represented the right strategy. By buying and holding stocks then paying in the top 30 percent of dividends, I would have helped my clients recover within just three and a half years.

All the other portfolios required more than a decade to come back to where they started.

Of course, if I *had* seen the Great Depression coming, I would certainly have done much better by moving my clients entirely out of the market and into cash. But I am a mere mortal—I cannot see the future.

Now, however, I can offer a clear direction for recovery from a crash. If you follow my investment strategy, based on Shiller's discovery, you should have no fear of a serious market tumble. You will know what to do.

Indeed, I used this precise strategy to help my clients recover rapidly from the crash of 2008.

Did I see 2008 coming? No. Did my clients pull out of the tailspin fast? Yes.

PUTTING SHILLER AND FAMA TOGETHER

The insights of Shiller and Fama may at first seem contradictory, but they are not. Fama essentially argues that the market won't become mispriced because of information. Shiller argues that when the market becomes mispriced, it's because of emotion.

In the right light, you can see these positions as two sides of the very same coin. And the net result of both positions is the same.

You cannot pick out one piece of information and use that piece of information to choose a stock or time the market. You cannot read an article from the *Wall Street Journal* or watch Jim Cramer's show and expect to beat the market.

If you follow the logic of either thinker, you will realize that if you chase the market, you are going to lose money. If you follow either thinker, you will see that the greatest danger facing you will be your own emotions. If you don't control your emotions, they will mirror the market, and the market will beat you.

BELIEVING IN SCIENCE

I said earlier that financial advisors often find physicians difficult to work with because physicians often have a hard time accepting advice. But after years of working with my physician clients, I have found that when it comes to investment science, we usually have a meeting of the minds.

I know when you prescribe a treatment to your patients, you will do so only if a body of clinical research backs up your decisions. You refuse to listen to hearsay, anecdotal evidence, or unreferenced statistics. I work the same way. When I show my physician clients the rigorous, independent, evidence-based investment studies performed in the academic world, they generally feel at home.

From here on, nobody's dog-and-pony show, however well performed, should ever impress you again. Not the antics of a soothsayer shouting from a TV studio, the promises of a Wall Street broker sitting in a mahogany-lined office, or the smile of a hedge fund manager lounging in the Hamptons.

Invest with science. Invest with confidence. Ignore the witch doctors.

In the next chapter, we'll see how good investing is only part of an overall *process* for wealth management. Then, we'll look at how to pick an honest advisor to complete that process.

CHAPTER SIX

The Process of Wealth
Management

The problem with most financial planning lies in the very
concept of a "plan."

Usually, when you engage a financial planner, you will write
a check for $3,000 or $4,000 minimum, turn over a list of
your assets and expenses, attend a couple of meetings, and
then you'll receive a detailed plan. This plan represents the
deliverable from the engagement, and everyone feels as if
they've done their job.

Your financial plan will be beautifully presented—probably
in a thick, embossed binder. It will have been generated
by a piece of software designed to spew out many, many
pages of charts and graphs, including a whole chapter
of disclaimers.

Most often, this plan proves not only difficult to read but also nearly impossible to carry out. Why? Not just because the approach was generic and cookie-cutter, but because just as health cannot be prescribed, neither can wealth.

Financial well-being is not achieved through a one-time plan, no matter how detailed and filled with charts. *Financial well-being is achieved by a rigorous, repeatable process practiced over many years.*

Within three weeks, something in every physician's situation will change. Within a few months, the original plan usually becomes just one more binder gathering dust on your office shelf—a binder that you do not read.

Only a *process* works over time.

THE GOALS OF A GOOD PROCESS

In Chapter 4, we learned about the six pillars of wealth management, and in Chapter 5, we took a close look at the most important pillar—wealth preservation or investment. Now, you need to understand the full process of wealth management, beginning with the realization that it involves a lot more than good investing.

You also need to understand the role of a financial advisor.

My own process for wealth management was developed through my participation in a remarkable roundtable of financial advisors—a roundtable that grew out of a workshop given by John Bowen. Bowen built two financial advisory firms, one worth $1.5 billion and one worth $25 billion. He did that by focusing on a process, but like me, he *assumes the use of a competent financial advisor*, someone who will both follow and manage the process for you.

The overall goal of my process is to relieve physicians of the drudgery of keeping their personal finances in good order. It recognizes that you will never have time to fully develop your own expertise in finance. That you have a hard enough time practicing medicine, keeping up with the changes in medical science, and of course, staying current with medicine's ever-shifting regulatory and administrative duties.

Not everyone needs a highly involved financial advisor with this kind of process in place. But I'm pretty sure you, as a physician, do. In this chapter, I lay out my personal process as a model for the process of working with *any* financial advisor.

INFORMATION AT ALL TIMES

My own wealth management process has been designed to understand a physician's financial picture, *not at one point in time but all of the time.* It's a method for ensuring that a financial advisor stays on top of the client's situation month in and month out. Only with this kind of total understanding can an advisor provide the best advice and solutions within the ever-changing circumstances of modern financial life.

In other words, a good advisor and a good client both recognize that planning rests on two constants: *change and the awareness of change.*

Awareness, of course, must go in both directions. Advisors like me do more than advise; we act on behalf of our clients. A good process must ensure that a client knows what the advisor is doing, when it's happening, and why.

Too often, clients do not understand or do not even know what their financial advisors, wealth managers, or investment brokers are up to with their money. With my process, I ensure that decisions are not just understood by my clients, but we stay on the same page as well.

Another information loop involves outside domain experts. No financial advisor has complete expertise in all aspects of wealth management—the six pillars we discussed in Chapter 4.

It's simply impossible for any one person to gather the

necessary knowledge in each of these areas and keep that knowledge up to date. In fact, most advisors have deep expertise in only one of the six pillars. My specialty, for example, is investments. I do not pretend to know enough about estate planning, tax law, or practice succession to fully advise my clients in these areas.

My process ensures that outside experts with supporting solutions are engaged when needed, and I monitor my clients' situation through a disciplined, ongoing information cycle.

ADVISORS VERSUS MANAGERS

As we explore the proper role of a financial advisor, I should pause to repeat my warning about the titles or "hats" that people in my profession wear: *advisor, planner, manager, agent, broker.*

Usually (but not always), people who call themselves *financial planners* do not manage assets on behalf of their clients. They tend to do planning and charge a one-time or hourly fee. They may be a Registered Investment Advisor (RIA), or they may not.

Financial advisors or wealth managers may manage their clients' assets and make investments on their behalf. If they are brokers, the assets are usually held in the brokerage firm that employs them. If they are independent RIAs, the assets are usually held by a third-party custodian.

People who call themselves wealth managers tend to work with wealthier clients. Financial advisors tend to work across a broader range of incomes.

But you will find no hard-and-fast rules. Let me emphasize again that such hats may be worn or removed at will.

For the sake of convenience, I will refer to everyone who both advises and acts on behalf of their clients as financial advisors. Just remember, you cannot be certain of anyone's precise role or way of doing business just from their title. You need to ask.

In Chapter 7, we will talk about how to choose a financial advisor, regardless of the hat he or she chooses to wear.

CUSTODY OF ASSETS

No doubt you noticed the important difference in the previous discussion between advisors who *hold* the assets of their clients and those merely *authorized to manage* those assets. The common word is *custody*, but the definition of that word remains unclear. An advisor may have *custody* whether the advisor actually holds the assets or not.

In my case, I have the authority to make investment decisions on behalf of my clients and to charge them a fee deducted from their assets. However, my clients' assets are not held by me directly; they are held by Fidelity Investments, an independent firm. I feel strongly that this is the proper arrangement between a client and a financial advisor, as it goes a long way toward preventing criminal activity.

The infamous Bernie Madoff both held the assets of his clients *and* made their investment decisions. That allowed him to keep two sets of books—one to show his clients and one to steal their money. Such a scam would have been impossible if a reputable third party had held the assets.

The overall message? Inquire closely about the specific custodial arrangements made by any financial advisor, regardless of his or her title or institutional affiliation, and choose an advisor who uses a third-party custodian with a solid reputation. The top two custodians in the United States are presently Charles Schwab and Fidelity Investments.

This advice may vary if you consider an in-house advisor at a large full-service brokerage firm like Merrill Lynch or Wells Fargo. You may perhaps elect to place your confidence in such an institution, even though they are acting as both your custodian and your broker, and even though their own motives may be mixed. (Remember, for example, the cautionary tale of Dr. Zuck.)

However, if you work with an *independent advisor*, make sure he or she is not both investing your money and holding it in his or her own accounts.

THE DISCOVERY MEETING

The process of wealth management begins with a carefully structured series of meetings with a prospective client, launched with the *discovery meeting*.

I need to discover the client, and the client needs to discover me. At this meeting, I ask a large number of questions, including philosophical inquiries such as, "What does money mean to you?"

I really do need to understand a physician's life goals, short and long term, if I am to help him or her reach those goals. I need to understand income and expenses, assets and liabilities, aspirations, interests, and hobbies. Many people are supporting their parents, disabled siblings, children with special needs, or children with drug problems. They're paying alimony or considering a speculation in a business. I will delve into a potential client's community engagement, charitable inclinations, church attendance—*everything*.

I ask about everything, because without understanding everything, I cannot really grasp a client's overall financial picture. Money really does touch every aspect of life.

In general, I break out my questions into the following categories.

- Values: How do you see money? What do you hope to accomplish with money?
- Goals: Long-term, short-term, personal, family, social, global
- Relationships
- Assets, liabilities, income, expenses, lifestyle, lifestyle aspirations
- Interests and hobbies

Other advisors the client may be working with: Are these advisors reactive or protective? What is their process?

Of course, I also encourage my clients to ask *me* a lot of questions—about my own past, my own goals, and my approach to financial management.

Because we are heading into a long-term process together, not into a one-time plan, the quality of our relationship will matter a great deal. We must get a gut feeling about each other.

Usually, by the end of such a meeting, I know whether I can provide substantial value to a prospective client, and I will only go to the next step if I think I can provide that value. If not, I will point them to other advisors, or simply ask them to read certain books.

The prospective client must also, of course, decide if they can work with me. Even more: *Will they enjoy working with me in a trust relationship?* If both sides decide to continue the exploration of the process and the relationship, we will move on to the next meeting.

RED FLAGS

Just about all financial advisors hold discovery meetings, although few go into sufficient depth with their prospective clients. We'll get to the questions you should ask at such a meeting in Chapter 7, but here are some red flags to watch out for.

The first red flag should be raised if a financial advisor tries to sell you a specific product at that first meeting, such as an annuity, an insurance plan, or a fund. It's way too soon for such a pitch to occur, and that should tell you that the "advisor" is really a salesperson.

The second red flag should be raised if the advisor does

not clarify the way in which they would take custody of your investments and the way in which they would report back to you or track your assets.

The third red flag should go up if your advisor seems to be too much of a lone wolf, working without outside experts. If someone pretends to have a deep understanding of tax law *and* investment strategy *and* estate planning, something is wrong.

In my own discovery meetings, I always spend a little time explaining the ecosystem of financial advising. If clients don't go with me, I want to make sure they don't make the grave mistake of falling into the hands of someone who does not have their best interests at heart.

In the chart, you will see an overview of the general process that should follow a discovery meeting with any good financial advisor.

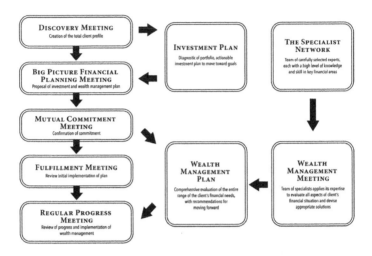

THE SECOND MEETING: BIG-PICTURE FINANCIAL PLAN

If a physician wishes to move forward after that first meeting, and I think it's a good fit, I will put together a big-picture plan to discuss at the *proposal meeting*.

It's a very simple plan, running about three pages, based on the six pillars of wealth management.

The first page gives a brief summary of the physician's situation as I understand it: monetary philosophy, goals, relationships, assets, liabilities, expenses, interests, hobbies, social engagement, charitable inclinations, and so forth.

The second page offers a high-level investment strategy

based on the summary in page one. Here, I lay out how much income I think the physician needs now and will need for retirement—along with supporting kids in school and paying off liabilities. This plan is based on the science we discussed in Chapter 5, but yes, it fits on one page.

The third page presents a wealth management action plan—the process of moving forward. Here, I include gaps I have seen in the physician's financial life that must be addressed. One doctor may be doing their own taxes each year and missing a lot of deductions. Another will have young children but has yet to do any planning on their behalf in case of his or her own death or incapacity.

In other words, this third page addresses each of the six pillars that will require expert help and will demand a long-term management process for the individual client. The expertise for each pillar will be found by me, as the "primary care physician," calling in specialists from my network as needed: a CPA, an estate attorney, a practice succession expert—whoever is needed.

I present my very short, three-page proposal at the second meeting. Physicians who have been handed thick binders by financial advisors in the past may be shocked, but most are relieved to see something immediately comprehensible and free of filler.

We go over the physician's feedback on the plan and see what needs to be adjusted. Then we size up our potential engagement together and discuss whether we want to move forward together. If your prospective financial advisor hands you a thick binder, ask him or her to summarize each section with simple words, and look at the underlying process and investment philosophy rather than the charts.

Sometimes a potential client will become very excited and want to sign up with me on the spot. But I don't want anyone to make a decision at this second meeting. I tell potential clients that such a decision involves a long-term relationship, and it is too important for any quick judgments. I tell them to sit on the proposal for a week or so and come back for a third meeting.

THE THIRD MEETING: COMMITMENT

Like many advisors, I call the third meeting a *mutual commitment meeting*. Some call it the onboarding meeting.

The cool-down period has passed. The plan has been adjusted, based on feedback from the second meeting. Papers have been prepared for an advisory agreement, which gives me authority to manage assets through a third-party custodian. The client will also sign papers with that third-party custodian, in my case Fidelity Investments, so that it will begin holding his or her assets.

If everything's a go, the physician has become a client.

THE FOURTH MEETING: FULFILLMENT

The fourth meeting, often called the fulfillment meeting, comes anywhere from two to four weeks later. At this point, I have begun moving the new client's money into the hands of my third-party custodian, and a number of investments will have been placed.

Now I need to sit down with the physician to explain what I have been up to, and how the process is moving forward.

It's not unusual to encounter a little nervousness at this point, maybe even some buyer's remorse. In spite of all our conversations, a physician may have woken up one morning and suddenly realized, *Hey, this guy is moving my money around. What's going on? Am I crazy to do this?*

Clients may have already received the first statements from the third-party custodian (again, in my case, Fidelity), and I need to teach them how to read those statements. At this point, I usually do provide a binder, but it's intended for keeping statements and other financial records properly organized. I ask the client to use that binder for everything and to make notes there with questions for our future meetings.

This fourth meeting always proves important and timely. It firmly establishes our working relationship, and it brings the physician fully into the loop.

REGULAR PROGRESS MEETINGS

After that important fourth meeting, I meet with my clients a minimum of once a quarter—more often, of course, if their situation is complex.

At these regular meetings, I will first report on what we have accomplished against the six pillars in the previous quarter, with an emphasis on investments. And then I will make sure I find out what has changed in the client's situation.

Life moves fast, and often I learn of previously unreported changes in a client's situation that require some action on my part—whether it be a new opportunity, a new goal, a new responsibility, or a potential danger.

Finally, we go back to my wealth management action plan, the third page of that three-page plan, and we decide on our priorities for the coming quarter.

Aside from the ongoing investment, or wealth preservation pillar, I try to focus actions on just one pillar per quarter, so that I do not overwhelm my client with actions and changes. Over the next quarter, we may focus on tax mitigation, in the next, we may work on practice succession, in the next, we might work on their heir protection, and so forth.

The regular progress meetings are the first repeatable loop in an iterative process.

BRINGING IN THE DOMAIN EXPERTS

After each regular progress meeting, I take the information I have gathered and loop in my domain experts. As I mentioned, these may include CPAs, attorneys, bankers, insurance experts, practice advisors, and other specialists. I will call a meeting with four or five of these people, sit down, and review the client's situation, including all the updates.

At these meetings, I'm looking for expert advice, forward actions, and warnings.

An attorney might say, "Wow, this doctor really needs to add such and such clause to his estate plan." The CPA might say, "She's not deducting a major expense, and she really needs to bring that into her accounting now so she can claim that deduction on April 15." A practice advisor might take a look at the work of an ENT and say, "This doctor is doing audiology, facial plastic surgery, immunization—a whole variety of work. But not all of these practices are equally profitable. Let's take a look and help him focus on the work that is the most profitable, instead of spreading himself so thin. Also, this doc really needs to bring in a younger associate, so he can begin planning for succession and retirement ten years from now."

Such experts see things I would not see, and they bring invaluable opinions and ideas to the big picture of the client's overall wealth—the picture that I must have as the "primary care physician" managing my client's financial health.

I will then bring these ideas and warnings to my client, so we can take action together. It's up to the client whether or not to use my recommended CPA, attorney, or other expert to implement these actions. They may choose to use their own expert, or do the work themselves. There's no obligation, but I do want to make sure the action occurs. I am only authorized to take *independent action* on my clients' investment portfolios.

FOCUS ON THE PROCESS

Both the regular progress meetings and the repeated loop

with the experts occur at least every quarter, and together, these two loops form the core of my approach to wealth management—not a single plan but *a relationship and a process.* By engaging in a similar process with a good financial advisor, your financial situation will improve year to year, with far fewer bumps in your fiscal road than you probably experience now.

The process requires discipline, it requires outside expertise, and it requires constant communication.

If you will forgive another health-care analogy, let me compare a sound financial process with regular exercise and a proper diet. A person does not become healthy and strong by going to the gym one time or eating one head of lettuce. A person becomes healthy and strong by going to the gym two or three days a week, every week, for their entire lives and by eating right day in and day out.

Here's a summary of the functions any good financial advisor must serve if he or she is to build the six pillars of your house of wealth:

- The financial advisor will use a consultative process to establish a close relationship with you in order to gain a detailed understanding of your values, needs, goals, resources, and obligations. *No cookie-cutter plans.*

- The advisor will coordinate a team of specialists who offer customized solutions designed to fit your specific needs. This team will take into account a range of interrelated financial services, such as investment management, insurance, retirement planning, estate planning, and business succession planning. *No lone wolves.*

- The advisor will deliver these customized solutions only in close consultation with you and will work closely with you on an ongoing basis to make sure all gaps and threats in your financial life are identified and addressed proactively. *You are always in the loop, and nothing is left out of the loop.*

In the next chapter, we'll talk about how to choose and interview an advisor who can help ensure your own financial health.

CHAPTER SEVEN

How to Choose a Financial Advisor

As I have mentioned many times, the only requirement for becoming a financial advisor is to call yourself a financial advisor. My mother, who is an Ob-Gyn and knows nothing about money, could call herself a financial advisor, and she would not be breaking any laws.

Generally speaking, however, only three types of people *tend* to call themselves financial advisors. Understanding their roles is the necessary first step to delegating your wealth management.

- Insurance agents: These could be captive agents, working for a single insurance company like New York Life or MetLife, or they could be independent agents who represent multiple insurance products. In either case, these folks make their living earning commissions from the insurance companies. They are under no obligation to disclose how much they make or how they make it. They are the insurance companies' agents; they are not your agents. *Still, their business card may read "financial advisor."*

- Stockbrokers: These folks may work for major Wall Street brokerages such as Goldman Sachs or Morgan Stanley, they may work for banks or other institutions, or they may work as an independent broker/dealer. Regardless, their job is to act as the middleman who facilitates transactions. *In other words, they earn money when transactions happen.* That makes them, at best, intermediaries. At worst, they may be counterparties who may actually be working against your interests. How much a stockbroker makes off you is their trade secret. They are certainly not your fiduciary. *But their business card may read "financial advisor."*

- Registered Investment Advisors (RIAs): These are the only "financial advisors" who are actually licensed to give financial advice. According to the law as of this writing, insurance agents and stockbrokers are not even allowed to give advice other than what is incidental to the products they sell.

RIAs are presently regulated by the Investment Advisors

Act of 1940, which requires them to undertake a fiduciary duty to their clients. By current law, they cannot accept third-party payments. They must also be completely transparent about their conflicts of interest, if any exist.

I call these *pure RIAs* to distinguish them from *hybrid RIAs*, who are RIAs who also have a broker license and/or an insurance license. They may even quietly operate these practices as separate companies. One company gives advice and then recommends you to the "other company" for your investment purchases, receiving two commissions on the same work.

I would prefer a hybrid RIA to a broker, but it's best to make sure your financial advisor (or wealth manager or financial planner or other expert) is a pure RIA, not a hybrid RIA. As of now, this at least means he or she is obligated by law to act in your best interest and that conflicts of interest are minimized.

In my experience, I do see a direct relationship between disclosure requirements and honor among financial advisors. In my opinion, fees and kickbacks should be disclosed, and advisors should indeed be required to act in the best interests of their clients.

As it stands, however, the situation is in flux, and you certainly cannot trust regulators to protect you. You need to make yourself personally aware of your advisor's *true* role in the financial world and his or her obligations to your financial well-being.

HOW TO INTERVIEW A FINANCIAL ADVISOR

Few financial advisors enjoy the level of education achieved by doctors. Regardless of their current expertise or commitment, however, many come from a background in sales. They tend to be highly social, talkative people, and they often appear "not serious" in the eyes of physicians. As I discussed in the introduction, physicians tend to be highly distrustful of financial advisors, to the point where many financial advisors actively avoid working with physicians.

As a result, many physicians end up handling their own finances—to their great detriment.

As a doctor, you need to bring your focus on facts and results to any business discussion, but I urge you to head into an interview with a potential advisor remembering the following truths: (1) You need someone doing this for you, (2) there *are* good people out there doing this, (3) expertise in financial matters does exist, and (4) you do not have time to build that expertise yourself.

With that attitude firmly in mind, you should approach the interview of a financial advisor as you would any employee. As this will be a long-term relationship, everything counts. Make the interview formal and comprehensive. Here's a breakdown of the areas you should consider. I call them the "Five C's"—character, chemistry, caring, competency, and cost-effectiveness.

CHARACTER

Make sure your financial advisor offers the highest level of integrity. That means he or she has not entered this profession just to make money but has a higher calling to help people. Often, this can be revealed simply by asking what brought the advisor to this kind of work. "I really get a rush from the stock market" may not be the best answer.

CHEMISTRY

Make sure you can connect with your financial advisor on an emotional level and that he or she "gets" you. Start out by engaging in a bit of small talk to see if your conversations flow naturally.

CARING

You need to get the sense that an advisor is genuinely concerned about your well-being. This is best determined by the questions *the advisor asks*, unprompted. Do they try to understand your current financial situation in all its aspects? Do they want to know your goals, dreams, aspirations, fears, and worries?

COMPETENCY

You need to ask some tough questions to ensure an advisor is technically capable. This means getting past the impressive charts and graphs you will be shown about past performance with other clients. Ask a few technical questions to see if he or she can answer them confidently. I suggest some later in this chapter. Also, see if they can discuss all six pillars of wealth management with some confidence.

During the interview, you will get a sense of the educational level achieved by the advisor. You may even want to inquire about that level. Again, you are unlikely to find someone who, like you, has completed many years of postgraduate education. But there are people out there acting as financial advisors who did not even complete high school.

COST-EFFECTIVENESS

Make sure the advisor delivers true value relative to cost. Most charge 1 percent on assets under management (AUM), and fees should not deviate too greatly from that. Some will offer discounts on larger portfolios. For example, an advisor may charge 1 percent on the first million in assets, then perhaps 0.7 percent on assets above $1 million up to $5 million, and 0.4 percent on everything beyond $5 million.

Remember, however, that brokers and insurance agents will receive additional kickbacks from fund companies. If they sell you a mutual fund or an insurance policy, the net cost to you may well double.

On investments wrapped in insurance policies, your "advisor" will be getting 3 percent or 3.5 percent above and beyond what they are charging you for advice. Not only does this represent a conflict of interest in their choice of investment vehicle, but you are absolutely paying fees you should not pay.

That means that over ten years, you can easily give up 35 percent of your wealth without even knowing it.

Truly, if you use an insurance agent as your investment advisor, it is very unlikely you can retire well, as most of your wealth will have been transferred to the insurance company by the time you retire. Not surprisingly, as the least regulated industry in finance, insurance extracts the most money.

A broker is a little better but not much. With a Wall Street broker, you will be paying about 2.5 percent or losing 25 percent over ten years.

SUGGESTED INTERVIEW QUESTIONS

Here are some suggested questions to ask a potential financial advisor. I am certain you will find the answers revealing. The questions are intentionally similar to questions an employer would ask a potential employee.

- *Do you have a Series 7 license?* The correct answer is *"no."* A Series 7 license is a broker license. Having this license means your advisor is actually a broker who can take third-party kickbacks without your knowledge.
- *Do you have a license to sell insurance policies?* Again, the correct answer is *"no."* You want a pure RIA as your financial advisor, not an insurance agent.
- *What license do you have?* The correct answer is *Series 65*. This is the RIA license that currently requires the holder to act as a fiduciary.
- How and when did you become a financial advisor? What brought you to the wealth management business? Here, you are looking for character: an honest desire to help people.
- Tell me your proudest moment as a financial advisor. Again, you are looking for character.

- I'm sure you do great work, but every road has bumps. Tell me about a moment in your work as a financial advisor that made you ashamed. This question can reveal a great deal—even if the advisor avoids answering it.
- *What do you enjoy most as a financial advisor?* You must judge for yourself if this answer resonates with you.
- *Who are your clients? Do you work with any particular niche or type of client?* Ideally, the advisor will have extensive and specific experience with physicians—but don't prompt for this.
- *Have you heard of Eugene Fama?* If the advisor has not heard of Eugene Fama, Nobel Prize winner and the father of modern finance, you should be very concerned. If you have read Chapter 5, you will know that this single question may be enough to reveal an advisor's knowledge base.
- *What is your investment philosophy?* Compare this against the brief summary I present at the end of Chapter 5. If an advisor cannot articulate a substantially similar philosophy, look elsewhere.
- *Who is on your team? What are the resources you rely on to do your job?* You must be sure your advisor is not operating alone but maintains a significant network of internal or external expertise. Again, don't prompt for the answer. Don't ask, "Do you pull in estate attorneys as needed?"

- *Tell me about your overall consultative process.* The advisor should be able to lay out a process similar to the one I outlined in Chapter 6. Indeed, the advisor should be focused on a process and not treat process as an afterthought. If you ask, "How often do we meet?" then the advisor should not reply, "As often as you like."
- *What aspects of wealth management do you help with?* Again, don't prompt with specifics. The advisor should be able to list categories similar to my six pillars.
- *What are your fees, and how are they structured and billed?* See "Cost-Effectiveness" above for a full discussion of proper fees.
- *Do you personally receive any commissions on transactions?* Remember that these are on top of fees and always represent a conflict of interest.
- *What do you see as the biggest value you provide to your clients?* This open-ended question should help you understand whether you are working with someone who provides a long-term wealth management process or is simply looking to place your investments and take in a fee.

ARE YOU DEALING WITH A MERE SALESPERSON?

After you have completed this interview, ask yourself, "Is this someone I can trust? Someone who will have my back? Someone I can call in a crisis?"

You don't want to work with a person whose advice will always leave you with a nagging doubt. In the good times, you may not worry about questionable advice or incomplete follow-through. In the good times, you may say to yourself, "OK, my doubts can be swept under the rug. My portfolio is going up. We have a great time playing golf together." But then, when the rough times come, you will have no one to trust, and no one you can rely on to take action.

Too often, a "financial advisor" is really a salesperson.

By asking these questions, I hope you can discover the truth behind the business card. But beyond determining competence and trustworthiness, you really do need to find out if the advisor *cares* about your outcomes. After the interview, ask yourself, "Does this person care? Will this person really try to understand my situation?"

Physicians often tell me about financial advisors who jumped right to "solutions" barely fifty minutes into their first conversation. By doing this, such advisors show they do not really care to understand a physician's full situation— they are just trying to sell the physician something. Fifty minutes is not enough time to grasp anyone's complete set of financial and personal issues, and certainly not those of a physician. The "solution" is usually a lucrative product with a high commission that the advisor is eager to close.

If the advisor is just a salesperson, his or her job will essentially be over once the product has been sold. The commission usually comes up front, and these salespeople know that once they gather your assets and score their commission, their time will be better spent on new clients. After that, every phone call with you that does not lead to an additional sale will just be a waste of their time, a cost of doing business. This is especially true of insurance salespeople, because brokers can often find ways to churn your stocks and score additional kickbacks on your portfolio.

Indeed, most of the training that "financial advisors" receive at a large brokerage like a Morgan Stanley has little to do with investment strategy and even less to do with wealth management. Most of the training really is in sales. Such institutions will recruit a bunch of young people and give them a list of two hundred numbers to call. "Cold call these numbers and try to schedule an appointment. You're playing a numbers game. The more calls, the more likely you will score. Get used to hearing no and moving on."

Afterward, the office will hold a group meeting and extol the person who made the most calls and scheduled the most meetings. I experienced this firsthand when I went to a recruiting meeting at a large brokerage.

By the time such training is over, these "advisors" have

become numb to rejection and to people saying no over and over again. Worse, they will have become accustomed to befriending people with the goal of selling them something. They will have learned to take people out for coffee, cultivate their trust, and then move a product. *That's their primary skill. And it's how they are evaluated.*

At the end of the month, these people are not asked, "Did you help your clients improve their financial situation?" They are asked, "Did you meet your production target? Did you gather enough money from your clients?"

Tax mitigation? Estate planning? Practice succession? Brokers generally learn little or nothing about such subjects. *Nevertheless, their business cards will often read "financial advisor."*

EDUCATED IN ALL SIX PILLARS

Earlier, I said that a good financial advisor cannot possibly offer sufficient expertise in all six pillars of wealth management. Nevertheless, like a primary care physician, he or she must be educated in all six pillars.

I regularly attend training seminars in accounting, law, estate planning, and other areas of concern to my clients. I know I need to pull in genuine expertise as needed, but

I make sure I am strong enough in each area that I can identify opportunities and pitfalls in my clients' situations.

For example, physicians will often own the buildings in which they practice; that makes them commercial real estate investors. As a financial advisor, I need to have enough understanding of commercial real estate tax law to see opportunities for savings and then bring in a CPA with the focused expertise.

My own primary expertise is investing, but another advisor may have a different primary expertise, such as accounting and tax law. Such an advisor must be sufficiently self-aware to call on outside experts in investing and not try to wing it.

Interview more than one potential financial advisor. Make sure each one can talk intelligently about all six pillars of wealth management. Make sure each knows their limitations.

And please, don't choose a *salesperson.*

Conclusion

THE ART OF DELEGATION

I have a client who is not a physician but a very successful banker. He founded one of the largest mortgage banks in Maryland, and I once asked him the secret to his success. He gave me an answer I will never forget:

"I picked the two or three things I'm really good at. The rest I delegated."

You will not find delegation in the work ethic of most people you meet, even the smartest. And doctors seem to have a special problem with the whole concept.

As I said in the introduction, this may come from the vital confidence any physician must have in their own judgment.

To do your work, you must honestly believe you know how to handle something within your specialty better than anyone.

Still, if you had a patient with an eye problem, you would insist they see an ophthalmologist. If you broke your wrist, you would not treat it yourself, but you would visit an orthopedist.

The real problem comes with things you *could* do yourself but really should not.

One of my clients is a primary care physician who sees patients for eight hours a day and then spends another three hours inputting patient information into an EMR system. He could use a medical scribe for this work, but he's not comfortable delegating.

It may be true that a scribe would not do as good a job as the doctor inputting the information. Especially in the beginning, the work might include some errors. But surely, this doctor could oversee the scribe's work, review the records, and the scribe would improve over time. Little by little, the doctor could liberate himself from three hours of unnecessary labor every single working day.

It's not just doctors, of course. Delegation may not be taught in medical schools, but it's rarely taught even in business schools. Indeed, I have heard it said by otherwise very intelligent friends, "If you don't delegate, you will always have a job." I am tempted to reply, "On the other hand, if you don't delegate, *you will only have a job.*"

The unspoken truth is that you cannot have a business or, for that matter, a life, without some delegation.

I think you will *always* find delegation in the work ethic of the most successful individuals.

Without your own effective delegation strategy for your personal finances, your efforts will always be spread too thinly, mistakes will always be made, and one of the six pillars of your financial house will always be neglected.

TAKING ACTION

If you have read this book, I hope I have convinced you of two things: every pillar of your financial house matters, and you cannot hold each pillar up alone.

As you are a physician, I can also talk frankly to you about *timeliness.*

If you had a patient sitting in your office with a long-term condition, something that had troubled them for years, you would not suggest that they ignore it for a few more years to see if it improves. You would ask them to take immediate action. If they felt a pain in their chest and had shortness of breath, you would not tell them to ignore it.

Your poorly placed investments are a long-term condition that requires immediate action. Your unwritten estate plan threatens your loved ones. That painful tax bill needs attention.

Take immediate action to get your personal finances in good order, but do it through delegation. As a result of reading this book, I hope you will immediately seek out a qualified, fee-only financial advisor to help you gain full control—not as a one-time event but as part of a long-term relationship and a disciplined, repeatable process.

You may have leads on advisors from other physicians. If not, you can start by looking at the website of the National Association of Personal Financial Advisors (NAPFA) at www.napfa.com. There, you can search for fee-only advisors in your local area.

If you like, you can learn more at my own website, www. mzcap.com, or e-mail me personally at mzhuang@mzcap. com. I will be happy to reply.

After that, you must of course do your due diligence, conduct your formal interview, and carefully gauge both trust and chemistry. Take this book with you to the meeting, and conduct your interview right out of Chapter 7.

I say that because, as much as we devote books and movies to the subjects of love, hate, greed, lust, and the like, *procrastination* may be the strongest human trait of all. A vague intention is not enough. Don't just think to yourself, *I'm really going to give an independent financial advisor a call at some point*. Often, "some point" never comes, especially if the task seems large and overwhelming.

Take concrete action now. Call me now, e-mail me, or schedule a meeting. At least put a firm date on your calendar when you will do any of the above.

After you have read this book, I'm hoping you will be the person who does make the call, sends the e-mail, or sets up the appointment with an independent advisor. Once you begin the process, your efforts will gain momentum, and bit by bit, you will build a strong financial house. Take the first step, and you are 50 percent there.

PHYSICIAN, HEAL THYSELF

I began this book with a story about how I got into the

business of helping physicians with their personal finances. I saw a good man who had devoted his life to the well-being of others but had never made basic provisions for the well-being of himself and his family.

Since that day, I have worked with many physicians and have seen up close the personal hurdles that come with one of the most important jobs on earth. It has been my privilege to help my clients overcome some of these hurdles, and over the years, I believe I have helped to lower the stress of their lives.

I hope that you have found this book useful in better understanding not just your finances but also your career, your challenges, and your opportunities.

May you continue to take care of others.

And may you never forget to take care of yourself.

About the Author

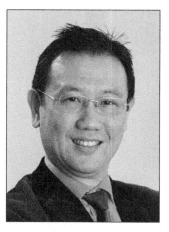

MICHAEL ZHUANG is founder and principal of MZ Capital Management, a financial advisory firm that focuses on wealth management for doctors. Previously, his career in investing included working with Société Générale, PG&E, and starting his own hedge fund. Michael holds dual master's degrees in mathematics and quantitative finance from Carnegie Mellon University. He blogs at The Investment Scientist and KevinMD and is a regular contributor to Morningstar, *Physician Practices*, and Investopedia, where he is recognized as a Top 100 Influential Advisor. In his spare time, Michael enjoys performing as a storyteller and stand-up comedian.